A surgeon's writing and publishing

Edited by

M. Schein, J. R. Farndon & A. Fingerhut

BJS

tfm Publishing Limited, Castle Hill Barns, Harley, Shrewsbury, Shropshire, SY5 6LX, UK

Tel:	+44 (0)1952 510061
Fax:	+44 (0)1952 510192
E-mail:	nikki@tfmpublishing.com
Web site:	www.tfmpublishing.com

Design and layout:	Nikki Bramhill BS (Hons) Dip Law
First Edition	September 2001
Reprinted	August 2006, September 2013
Paperback	ISBN-10: 1-903378-01-X
	ISBN-13: 978-1-903378-01-4

E-book editions:	February 2013
ePub	ISBN: 978-1-903378-87-8
Mobi	ISBN: 978-1-903378-88-5
Web pdf	ISBN: 978-1-903378-89-2

Acknowledgement

Some of the material within this book has been reproduced from the *British Journal of Surgery* with the kind permission of the publisher, © 2000 Blackwell Science Ltd.

2000, 87 (1) 3-5; 2000, 87 (2) 132-134; 2000, 87 (3) 261-264; 2000, 87 (4) 388-389; 2000, 87 (5) 532-533; 2000, 87 (6) 691-692; 2000, 87 (7) 835-836; 2000, 87 (8) 980-982; 2000, 87 (9) 1123-1124; 2000, 87 (10) 1284-1286; 2000, 87 (11) 1444-1447; 2000, 87 (12) 1603-1604; 2000, 87 (12), 1605-1609; 2000, 87 (12) 1610-1614.

Contents

Page Number

Chapter 1   1
Why should a surgeon publish?
M. Schein, J. R. Farndon and A. Fingerhut
Commentary by U. Schöeffel

Chapter 2   11
What should surgeons write?
P. R. O'Connell
Commentary by R. C. G. Russell

Chapter 3   21
Where can the surgeon publish?
M. Schein and A. Fingerhut
Commentary by J. L. Meakins

Chapter 4   33
Generating an idea: will it be publishable?
M. G. Sarr
Commentary by N. O'Higgins

Chapter 5   53
On getting started
D. Alderson
Commentary by N. S. Williams

Chapter 6   63
Writing a manuscript
S. A. Wells Jr.
Commentary by D. M. Dent

Contents

	Page Number

Chapter 7   73
Advice on writing style
J. R. Farndon
Commentary by W. B. Campbell

Chapter 8   87
The 'foreign' author
M. Rothmund and A. Fingerhut
Commentary by R. Saadia

Chapter 9   95
Essential statistics
G. D. Murray
Commentary by B. C. Reeves

Chapter 10   107
Writing about a surgical technique
A. Hirshberg and K. L. Mattox
Commentary by A. Darzi

Chapter 11   115
The final product
J. A. Murie
Commentary by A. E. Young

Chapter 12   125
What an editor wants or expects from authors
C. H. Organ
Commentary by A. L. Warshaw

Chapter 13   133
How to write a chapter
A. Fingerhut
Commentary by M. W. Büchler

Page Number

Chapter 14   143
How to edit or write a book
M. Schein
Commentary by L. M. Nyhus

Chapter 15   159
How to write a commentary
A. Fingerhut

Chapter 16   163
On the editor's desk
J. R. Farndon and J. A. Murie
Commentary by A. E. Baue

Chapter 17   175
Politics in surgical publishing
C. J. Laitman and L. F. Rikkers
Commentary by M. W. Büchler

Chapter 18   185
Dealing with the rejected article
P. J. Guillou and J. J. Earnshaw
Commentary by R. E. Condon

Chapter 19   193
Research misconduct:
diagnosis, treatment and prevention
M. J. G. Farthing
Commentary by G. M. Stirrat

Chapter 20   213
Internet communication and e-publishing
W. D. Neary and J. J. Earnshaw
Commentary by R. Smith

Contents

Page Number

Epilogue   223
Key considerations in surgical publishing
M. Schein, J. R. Farndon and A. Fingerhut

Appendix I   235
Guidelines on good publication practice
Committee on Publication Ethics (COPE)

Appendix II   251
Improving the quality of reports of meta-analyses of
randomised controlled trials: the QUOROM statement
The QUOROM Group

Appendix III   269
The CONSORT statement: revised recommendations
for improving the quality of reports of parallel-group
randomised trials
The CONSORT Group

Appendix IV   285
Consensus statement on submission and
publication of manuscripts

Contributors

D. Alderson MD FRCS, Professor of GI Surgery, Bristol Royal Infirmary, Bristol, UK.

A. E. Baue MD, Professor Emeritus of Surgery, Vice President for the Medical Center, Emeritus, Saint Louis University School of Medicine, St. Louis, Missouri, U.S.A.

M. W. Büchler MD, Professor of Surgery, Chairman, Department of General Surgery, University of Heidelberg, Heidelberg, Germany.

W. B. Campbell MS FRCP FRCS, Consultant Surgeon and Honorary Professor, Royal Devon and Exeter Hospital, Exeter, UK.

R. E. Condon MD MSc FACS, Professor and Chairman, Emeritus, Department of Surgery, The Medical College of Wisconsin, Milwaukee, U.S.A.

A. Darzi MD FRCS FRCSI FACS, Professor of Surgery, Academic Surgical Unit, St. Mary's Hospital, London, UK.

D. M. Dent ChM FRCS (Eng) FCS (SA), Professor of Surgery, Head of Department. Department of Surgery, Faculty of Health Sciences, University of Cape Town, Cape Town, South Africa.

J. J. Earnshaw DM FRCS, Consultant Surgeon, Gloucestershire Royal Hospital, Gloucester, UK.

J. R. Farndon BSc MD FRCS, Professor and Head of Division, University of Bristol and Consultant Surgeon, Bristol Royal Infirmary, Bristol, UK.

M. J. G. Farthing MD FRCP, Professor of Medicine, Faculty of Medicine, University of Glasgow, Glasgow, UK.

A. Fingerhut FACS, FRCPS (g) Chief of Service, Digestive Surgery, Centre Hospitalier Intercommunal, Poissy, France and Associate Professor of Surgery, Louisiana State University Medical School, New Orleans, LA, U.S.A.

P. J. Guillou BSc MD FRCS FRCPS (Glas) Hon, FMedSci, Dean of the School of Medicine, University of Leeds and Professor of Surgery, St. James's University Hospital, Leeds, UK.

A. Hirshberg MD, Associate Professor of Surgery, Michael E. DeBakey Department of Surgery, Baylor College of Medicine, Houston, Texas, U.S.A.

C. J. Laitman PhD, Senior Editor and Managing Editor, Annals of Surgery, University of Wisconsin Medical School, Clinical Science Center, Madison, Wisconsin, U.S.A.

K. L. Mattox MD FACS, Professor and Vice Chairman, Michael E. DeBakey Department of Surgery, Baylor College of Medicine, Houston, Texas, U.S.A. and Chief of Staff and Chief of Surgery, Ben Taub General Hospital, Houston, Texas, U.S.A.

J. L. Meakins OC MD FRCSC, Archibald Professor of Surgery, McGill University, Montreal, Canada.

J. A. Murie MA BSc MD FRCSEd FRCSG, Consultant Vascular Surgeon and Honorary Senior Lecturer, Department of Vascular Surgery, Royal Infirmary of Edinburgh, Edinburgh, UK.

G. D. Murray MA Dip Math Stat PhD CStat FRCP (Edin), Professor of Medical Statistics and Head of Public Health Sciences, Department of Community Health Sciences, University of Edinburgh Medical School, Edinburgh , UK.

W. D. Neary MB ChB MRCS, Vascular Research Fellow, Gloucestershire Royal, Hospital, Gloucester, UK.

L. M. Nyhus MD FACS, Warren H. Cole Professor and Head of the Department of Surgery, Emeritus, University of Illinois College of Medicine, Chicago, U.S.A.

P. R. O'Connell MD FRCSI, Consultant Surgeon, Mater Misericordiae Hospital, Dublin, Ireland.

N. O'Higgins MB BCh BAO MCh FRCS (Irl) FRCS (Eng) FRCS (Edin), Senior Professor of Surgery, University College Dublin, St. Vincent's University Hospital, Dublin, Ireland.

C. H. Organ Jr. MD FACS FRCSSA FRACS, Professor and Chairman, Department of Surgery, University of California-San Francisco, Oakland, California, U.S.A.

B. C. Reeves D Phil, Senior Lecturer in Epidemiology, Health Services Research Unit, London School of Hygiene and Tropical Medicine, London, UK.

L. F. Rikkers MD FACS, A. R. Curreri Professor and Chairman, Department of Surgery, University of Wisconsin Medical School, Clinical Science Center, Madison, Wisconsin, U.S.A.

M. Rothmund MD FACS FRCS (Eng), Professor and Chairman, Department of Surgery, Philipps-University, Marburg, Germany.

R. C. G. Russell MS FRCS, Chairman of the BJS Society and Consultant Surgeon, The Middlesex Hospital, London, UK.

R. Saadia MD FRCS (Ed), Charles William Burns Professor of Trauma Surgery, The University of Manitoba, Winnipeg, Manitoba, Canada.

M. G. Sarr MD, Professor of Surgery, Mayo Clinic, Rochester, Minnesota, U.S.A.

M. Schein MD FACS FCS (SA), Professor of Surgery, Cornell University Medical College and Bronx Lebanon Hospital, New York, U.S.A.

U. Schöeffel MD, Associate Professor of Surgery, Department of Surgery, University Hospital Freiburg, Freiburg, Germany.

R. Smith CBE BSc MB ChB FRCP FRCPE FFPHM FGAEK FRCGP FAMS FRCSE, Editor, BMJ and Chief Executive of the BMJ Publishing Group, BMJ editorial, London, UK.

G. M. Stirrat MA MD FRCOG, Emeritus Professor of Obstetrics & Gynaecology, and Senior Research Fellow in Ethics in Medicine, Centre for Ethics in Medicine, University of Bristol, Bristol, UK.

A. L. Warshaw MD, W. Gerald Austen Professor of Surgery, Harvard Medical School, and Surgeon-in-Chief and Chairman, Department of Surgery, Massachusetts General Hospital, Boston, U.S.A.

S. A. Wells Jr. MD, Professor of Surgery, Duke University School of Medicine, DUMC, Durham, NC, U.S.A.

N. S. Williams MS FRCS, Professor of Surgery, Director, Academic Department of Surgery, The Royal London Hospital, London, UK.

A. E. Young MA MChir FRCS, Consultant Surgeon, St. Thomas' Hospital, London, UK.

You are familiar with the wisdom of 'publish or perish' and you perceive that it might be advisable for you to follow this maxim but you do not know how to begin. Your senior colleagues press you to write but do not provide you with sufficient guidance. Perhaps your first language is not English and you are daunted by the prospect of working in the accepted language of academic science. Having been in your shoes only a few years ago the editors of this book know exactly how you feel. Let 'A surgeon's guide to writing and publishing' be your guide.

This book will tell you:

◆ Why it is good for you to write and publish.
◆ What you should write and publish.
◆ Where you should publish and about the differences between journals; how to choose the right venue for your publication.
◆ How to generate an idea and decide whether it is publishable.
◆ How to get started and write the manuscript.
◆ How to describe a surgical technique.
◆ What style to use.
◆ About Essential statistics.
◆ About the final product and what an editor expects from authors.
◆ What special precautions you need as a 'foreign' author.
◆ What happens with your paper after it lands on the Editor's desk and how to cope with rejections.
◆ About Politics and ethical issues in surgical publishing.
◆ About Internet and e-publishing and how to edit or write a book or a chapter.

The contributors to this book are leading surgical authors, many of whom are editors of renowned surgical journals.

After reading this book you should be better informed and successful in writing, publishing and editing. You will be ready to 'publish and not be damned'.

The Editors
September 2001

Chapter 1

Why should a surgeon publish?

M. Schein

Professor of Surgery, Cornell University Medical College & Bronx Lebanon Hospital, New York, U.S.A.

J. R. Farndon

Professor and Head of Division, University of Bristol & Consultant Surgeon, Bristol Royal Infirmary, Bristol, UK.

A. Fingerhut

Chief of Service, Digestive Surgery, Centre Hospitalier Intercommunal, Poissy, France & Associate Professor of Surgery Louisiana State University Medical School New Orleans, LA, U.S.A.

'Writing was everything' **Alfred Kazin.**

For the majority of surgeons writing is not everything and some will not write at all during their career. Exhausted by attempts at alleviating suffering and the increasingly difficult tasks of bread-winning and administrative duties, most surgeons will leave writing for others. We know, however, that there are many surgeons 'out there' who are young and eager to write, but do not have the slightest idea how to begin. If you are an established academic surgeon, this book may not be for you.

This book is, however, aimed at surgeons who have that novel idea, observation or message waiting to be published but do not know the route leading to successful publication (and thereby dissemination) in the pages of a surgical journal. You wish to share a valuable experience with the rest of the surgical world but there is no one to guide you.

Some 'How to Write/Publish' books for scientists and medical professionals are available but to date none has ever been dedicated to surgeons. We intend to attempt to do this in each chapter of the book by providing insight into a range of different topics. We intend to be simple and brief, and to use practical examples from daily life. We sincerely hope that after reading this book you will be ready to write your own scientific or clinical surgical papers; not those that are regularly rejected but those that will be published in reputable journals.

Why should a surgeon publish?

'Reading maketh a full man, conference a ready man and writing an exact man.' **Francis Bacon**.

The reasons for writing and publishing are both egoistic and altruistic (Table 1). Being altruistic may eventually influence your ego as well!

TABLE 1
Why should a surgeon publish?

Egoistic motives	Altruistic motives
Academic promotion	Dissemination of knowledge
Professional promotion	Research selectivity*
Improve knowledge and judgement	
Being 'famous'	
Develop professional contacts	
Financial gain	

*   *Research selectivity is the process of fund allocation on quality of research to Universities in the UK.*

Egoistic motives for writing and publishing

Academic promotion

The dictum of 'publish or perish' is still firmly entrenched in academia. It is difficult to climb the academic ladder without a certain number of papers on your curriculum vitae. To progress academically to whatever academic title you aspire, your published output must constantly grow in number and quality. Obviously publications are not the only key to promotion but, as Bulwer-Lytton said, 'The pen is mightier than the sword'. In some countries, the number and quality of publications (graded on where the paper was published and how many times it has been cited) have a direct influence on academic ascension.

Professional promotion

This commonly follows academic promotion and vice versa. Let us say you are a resident or registrar seeking a prestigious fellowship or additional training in a centre of excellence, then your chances of competing successfully may be much better if only two to four relatively minor papers decorate your curriculum vitae. The mere fact that you have written and published signals to your potential employers that you are a 'thinker', interested in what you do and eager to share your experience with others. It will also suggest that you will continue to contribute academically in your new position. Do understand that writing and publishing is not limited to the 'academic surgical world'. Excellent and pioneering papers were and still are produced by astute clinicians from the non-academic surgical community. Well published 'non-academic' surgeons are respected by their peers, and publications add stature to their personalities and professional respectability. Who will you tend to believe: the surgeon who has published her results in a respectable journal or the one who rises at a meeting and says, 'I did 100 such cases with excellent results but I simply never found time to write and publish'?

Improve knowledge and judgement

Most of the authors in this book will have separately published 100-200 articles each. Any such paper written and published, be it a case report or a prospective randomized trial, contributed to, and added depth to, knowledge and understanding of the topic around which the publication revolved. The process also widens and deepens your own acumen, and the more you know the better you can serve your patients and yourself. You will never forget a topic about which you have written. Horace said, 'The secret of good writing is sound judgement', but good writing also provides you with the judgement. It allows you to analyse what you did, reflect on it and do better the next time.

Being 'famous'

As John Kenneth Galbraith said, 'Authorship of any sort is a fantastic indulgence of the ego'. The satisfaction one feels seeing a name in print is human and so is the pleasure derived from being quoted by others. A well published surgeon soon becomes 'famous': not only a prophet in his home town but perhaps worldwide. You could be the best surgeon in town but only after your results are published will you also be recognized in the capital and beyond.

Don't we all want to be 'significant' in one way or another? As surgeons we achieve a certain measure of significance through healing. But the subjects we heal are temporary residents on earth. Publishing, if 'significant', may provide us with the sense of the much desired 'significant permanence'. Would anyone remember today the name of Rudolf Nissen had he not published? [1] As Emerson wrote, 'He that writes to himself writes to an eternal public'.

Develop professional contacts

'The universal object of men of letters is reputation,' said John Adams. The more you write the greater will be your reputation, which in turn makes you attractive to people of reputation across the world. The international professional contacts which develop increase your perspective and ability to publish, and become the basis for further exchanges and improvement of the quality of your work. The Medical Club is truly international with no joining requirements and no membership fees. The bonds of international friendship through authorship and the medical profession are strong and enriching of life itself.

Financial gain

'Money, money, all is money! Could you write even a penny novelette without money to put heart in you?' wrote George Orwell.

This, however, is not exactly true for the writing surgeon. Promotion and fame, which come with 'being well published', may eventually help you to acheive a better-paid position. But practically speaking, the time spent writing, if dedicated to fee-paying clinical work, would be much more profitable. Satisfaction, however, cannot always be measured in currency!

Altruistic motives for writing and publishing

'You don't write because you want to say something; you write because you've something to say,' wrote Scot Fitzgerald. This is also the main reason for you to write - to share your finding, experience and thoughts with the surgical community. The main purpose of professional publishing is to disseminate knowledge. What exactly should be written and published are the subject of further chapters in this book. All we need to mention here is that surgeons have a certain degree of moral obligation to publish any significant novel observation, be it 'positive' or 'negative', a 'success' or 'failure'.

In some national academic settings, research output and quality are measured and these measures play upon the amount of resource given by government to the university or college. Your productivity therefore feeds directly on to the financial well-being of your institution. Such a model is the Research Assessment Exercise in the UK. In some institutes research productivity and publishing activity are measured, and will determine proportions of your salary.

The pressures to publish are sometimes inordinate. We would like to think that publishing misdemeanours are mainly due to these pressures. We acknowledge that other factors may play a part in this process which causes inconvenience, embarrassment and undue work in those searching catalogues or indices. Readers will have seen the firm stance taken by the *British Journal of Surgery* (*BJS*), for example, on these issues and the editors of the *BJS* are committed members of the Committee on Publication Ethics (COPE). We are pleased to publish the COPE guidelines which can be located in Appendix I.

Not everyone shares these sentiments and there are those who think that there are too many journals and too many 'non-significant' publications. Some suggest limiting surgical output to a few top journals, 'supplied' by top academicians [2]. We contend, however, that such a non-egalitarian publishing world, if ever allowed to prevail, would produce a false and biased image of surgical practice, and show surgery as practised in highly sophisticated ivory towers. That surgical writing should not only be limited to a few aristocrats is reflected today on the Internet, as more surgeons flock to its surgical sites in order to learn and share experience and knowledge [3]. It appears obvious to us that many surgeons have something to say and there is a need to show them how to say it in peer-reviewed journals. We thought this task so important to deserve these precious pages into a full book publication; we know there are many of you across the world who always wanted to publish but did not know how. We hope this book will help you get started.

'All you ever wanted to know about (publishing) but never dared to ask' - modified from **Woody Allen**!

References

1   Schein M, Schein H, Wise L. Rudolf Nissen: the man behind the fundoplication. *Surgery* 1999; 125: 347-53.

2   Silen W. Publish or perish revisited. *Arch Surg* 1996; 131: 798.

3   Gilas T, Schein M, Frykberg E. A surgical Internet discussion list (Surginet): a novel venue for international communication among surgeons. *Arch Surg* 1998; 133: 1126-30.

Commentary
by U. Schöeffel
Associate Professor of Surgery, Department of Surgery, University Hospital Freiburg, Freiburg, Germany.

A surgeon´s guide to the world of publishing unquestionably has to start with reflections on motivations. The collection of egoistic and altruistic motives presented by the editors of this series seems almost complete and the expertise of the contributors is obvious, all of them having enriched the surgical literature. The reader may wonder whether it was the wish for increased reputation in the scientific community; the desire for personal satisfaction by writing to an 'eternal public'; or the pressure of a deeply felt moral obligation to disseminate knowledge and significant observations which served as the driving force behind such a tremendous amount of work.

In this context it may seem inadequate and cavilling to paraphrase the title by asking 'when (why) should a surgeon NOT publish'. However for those of us who have contributed relatively few ideas, observations, or messages to the field of written surgical evidence, some reflective thoughts may be appropriate.

For a surgeon, writing is not everything. Care for the patient, administrative duties, and teaching may indeed distract from proper research. The time spent at the writing desk may be too short to result in high quality articles. It has recently been suggested that as much as half of the research surgeons undertake is misconceived [1]. The common practice of granting publication of papers presented at regional meetings adds to a less than desirable overall quality of many surgical journals. As long as the publish or perish mentality prevails and impact factors matter, things will not change. But why should they change? To improve the bad reputation of surgical science? Or, even more important, to spare the precious time of fellow surgeons attracted by interesting titles or by keyword-search to articles the mediocrity of which may become disclosed only after reading the first few pages?

The responsibility remains with the authors. They have to assure the quality of submissions. Originality, importance, and scientific significance are the criteria to judge the value of an experience which one may want to share with the surgical community. Editors and reviewing peers may be of some help.

References

1   Horton R. Surgical research or comic opera: questions but few answers. *Lancet* 1996; 347: 984.

Chapter
1 ————————————————————————————————

Chapter 2

What should surgeons write?

P. R. O'Connell

Consultant Surgeon

Mater Misericordiae Hospital

Dublin, Ireland

George Bernard Shaw, writing on education, quipped that 'those that can do; those that cannot teach', to which an aggrieved headmaster added 'and those that can neither do nor teach, write'. While this exchange may hold a kernel of truth, it cannot apply in medicine and to surgery in particular. Of all the disparate subspecialties of medicine, surgery is for the doers, a craft as well as a science. Surgeons are the technicians of medical science. They have learnt by apprenticeship and experience but also by study of the rich library of surgical knowledge that has been handed down by previous generations. Word of mouth and anecdotal reference have not advanced surgical science or surgical techniques. Surgeons have relied on lucid, well illustrated and, in the modern era, peer reviewed information for education and governance. The challenge today is how to maintain this ethos of doing, teaching and writing at a time of rapid technological change, electronic communication and multimedia presentation.

The first stimulus - case report

The question 'What should I write?' is most often asked by a basic surgical trainee of a senior colleague when it is realized that career advancement dictates a minimum level of academic achievement, best measured by published work. It can be a daunting challenge for, in order to write, one must have information to convey, and both an ability to write and a suitable forum in which to get published. It follows that what to write depends on the opportunity that presents for writing. Frequently, the first stimulus for a young surgeon is an interesting patient who has prompted a literature search and perhaps a presentation to a local meeting. Many esteemed surgical writers, even journal editors, began a literary career with a time honoured case report [1]. Sadly, pressure on journal space and editorial policies directed at enhancing journal impact factor have reduced the opportunities for publication of case reports. None the less the writing of an interesting case report is a good start. It encompasses all of the elements that are part of the scientific publishing process:

observation; literature review; writing (and rewriting!); internal editing and external review. An original observation, such as that of mandibular swelling by Denis Burkitt and reported in *BJS* [2], can lead to important later discoveries and a lifetime interest in research.

Institutional review

The opportunity to review an individual unit or institutional experience of a particular condition or surgical procedure in a case series or cohort study, frequently presents during surgical training. This may be a trainee's first literary venture or the next step in surgical writing to follow publication of a case report [3]. The exercise is important since it can provide insight into the process and difficulties of surgical audit. Such retrospective data are more often of local interest but sometimes are of national or international importance and worthy of publication. Editors, guided by the peer review process, will require evidence of the importance of such data, often asking 'Is there anything new or important here?' The target readership of the particular journal will be of prime importance in making this decision.

Editors are increasingly wary of institutional databases that can be looked at in many ways and on many occasions. This is not to say that retrospective audit is not useful in moulding clinical practice. 'Salami slicing' of data is, however, to be discouraged. One good paper in a prestigious journal is worth many lesser publications. The concept of dividing a body of work into a large number of 'least publishable units' is well known but in practice it diminishes the value of the work and the reputation of the author.

Technical vignette

Technical innovation is always a topic of interest and the evolution of surgical technique depends much on individual ingenuity and perseverance. The extraordinary story of Edoardo Bassini, his revolutionary treatment of inguinal hernia [4], and subsequent description of his technique [5], exemplify surgical innovation, illustration and writing. More recently, descriptions of novel techniques such as fashioning an everted ileostomy [6], carotid arterial reconstruction [7] and laparoscopic cholecystectomy [8] are examples of innovation that have universally changed surgical practice. While most surgeons are from time to time tempted to cry 'eureka', few are blessed with the inspiration that leads to useful clinical application. Publication requires not just an idea, but evidence that the innovation is safe, of clinical value and widely applicable.

Laboratory based research

Surgical science takes as its foundation the formulation of a surgically relevant hypothesis that is tested in an experimental model. The majority of surgeons in training will undertake some period of formal laboratory or clinical research. This process, often in pursuance of a higher degree, can be a rich source of academic presentation and publication. A successful research project starts with a well-written experimental protocol that in turn provides a footplate on which to build subsequent scientific manuscripts. Every seasoned researcher knows that time spent in preparation of the protocol is time saved in writing a subsequent manuscript. Publication is an integral part of the experimental process that permits peer review and external recognition. A typical period of research may present opportunities to publish a new methodology, results of animal or clinical experiments and possibly a review article. It is in this period of training that most surgeons learn the discipline of surgical writing. Preparation, scientific method, data analysis and insightful discussion are integral parts of this process. Those fortunate enough will have as their academic supervisor a colleague with a keen sense of how and what to write. Others have to learn the discipline from the sometimes harsh rigours of the review process, or the sweeping changes required by an editor at the point of a red pen.

Scientific presentation

Presentation to a scientific meeting is the usual prelude to a scientific manuscript. The peer review process for abstract selection and constructive interchange with others of similar research interest allows selection of appropriate material for publication and facilitates discussion in the subsequent manuscript. The fact that there are many times more abstracts published than original articles illustrates how difficult it is to complete this process and how rigorous peer review can be. Because of this, prominent surgical journals, *BJS* included, attach particular importance to original articles emanating from certain surgical and scientific meetings, e.g. The Association of Surgeons of Great Britain and Ireland and The Surgical Research Society. Support of the British Journal of Surgery Society for this process is evidenced by sponsorship of *BJS* prizes at meetings of affiliated surgical societies.

Clinical trials

The outcome of a basic laboratory or clinical experiment may justify observation in a prospective clinical study and ultimate scrutiny in a randomized clinical trial. The importance of this process is evident from the prominence given by the *BJS* and other journals to randomized clinical trials. Organization of a randomized clinical trial is usually possible only in a large academic institution or national or international organization, but participation in multicentre trials is within the competence of most surgical units. In this situation, surgeons must be part of the scientific process of hypothesis generation, data collection, and analysis and publication. It is the latter elements of the process that are most easily delegated, but only surgeons should analyse and discuss those findings that are relevant to clinical surgery. The reporting of such should not be left to others. Evidence-based medicine has emerged as a discipline of clinical audit and governance. The Cochrane collaboration and others now compile clinical trial information. The Audit Commission now guides decisions concerning Government funding of clinical practice. These facts highlight the need for surgeons to be intimately involved in the scientific scrutiny that is now being applied to the discipline of surgery.

Review article

Review articles are an important part of the surgical literature occupying a middle ground between active research and established text. The relatively short time to publication of a journal review compared with a book chapter allows current literature to be compiled and interpreted in a manner that serves to educate and update the journal readership. Systematic review and meta-analysis have become important resources for health care providers and other decision-makers [9]. Such reviews are frequently written by other (non-surgeon) professionals. Surgeons should not neglect this part of their scientific responsibility, the importance of which is evident from the prominence they are accorded in the *BJS* and other journals.

Editorial

Topical or contentious issues in surgery may be dealt with in an editorial or leading article. These are usually written by invitation and place a burden of responsibility on the writer to review a subject objectively in a concise and impartial manner, ending with a conclusion that the reader can feel has the imprimatur of the journal's editorial board. An opportunity to write a leading article is not commonly afforded to a surgeon in training; nevertheless, a letter to the editor allows an opinion on recently published work or current issues to be aired. How the emergence of electronic publishing will alter journal correspondence remains to be seen. Most major journals, *BJS* included, have established or are in the process of establishing an interactive web-site on which active correspondence is encouraged.

Book chapter

The emergence of electronic publishing and CD-ROM text may change the medium in which book chapters and review articles appear. The possibility of including multimedia examples of surgical technique greatly enhances educational value, but these changes will not alter the essential need that surgeons have for ready access to up-to-date textbooks and detailed subspecialty reviews. Indeed, all practising surgeons will have a number of favourite texts to which they will occasionally revert. Some such texts are excellent examples of the various styles of surgical writing. The complexity of modern surgery is such that monographs are few and most such texts are multiauthored. Nevertheless the skills and vigilance of the editor are usually sufficient to ensure uniformity of style and excellence of content. The opportunity to contribute to such texts is both a professional challenge and a privilege that should not be delegated except under strict supervision.

Conclusion

The writing of prose does not always transfer to scientific surgical writing. The essence of scientific writing is to distil the subject matter to its core and then, confident of the fundamental hypothesis, expand to convince the readership of the case. The surgeon in training who poses the question 'what should I write?' faces a daunting challenge. There are many formats from which to choose. An impulse to write is a better start than a perceived need to write for career advancement. There is a discipline that has to be learnt and a style that has to evolve. Do not be afraid to start. Colleagues and even journal editors are there to help. Write as the opportunity allows. Above all, write what you as a surgeon would want to read.

References

1   Farndon JR, Taylor RM. Another rectal foreign body! *J R Coll Surg Edinb* 1978; 23: 96-7.

2   Burkitt D. A sarcoma involving the jaws in African children. *Br J Surg* 1958; 46: 218-23.

3   Hennessy TPJ, O'Connell R. Surgical treatment of squamous cell carcinoma of the oesophagus. *Br J Surg* 1984; 71: 750-1.

4   Thorwald J. Bassini. In: *The Triumph of Surgery*. London: Thames and Hudson, 1960: 274-95.

5   Wantz GE. The operation of Bassini as described by Attilio Catterina. *Surg Gynecol Obstet* 1989; 168: 67-80.

6   Brooke BN. The management of ileostomy, including its complications. *Lancet* 1952; ii: 102-4.

7   Eastcott HHG, Pickering GW, Rob CG. Reconstruction of internal carotid artery in a patient with intermittent attacks of hemiplegia. *Lancet* 1954; ii: 994-6.

8   Perissat J, Collet DR, Belliard R. Gallstones: laparoscopic treatment, intracorporeal lithotripsy followed by cholecystostomy or cholecystectomy - a personal technique. *Endoscopy* 1989; 21 (Suppl. 1): 373-4.

9   Moher D, Cook DJ, Eastwood S, Olkin I, Rennie D, Stroup DF. Improving the quality of meta-analyses of randomised controlled trials: the QUORUM statement. *Lancet* 1999; 354: 1896-900.

Commentary
by R. C. G. Russell

Chairman of the BJS Society and Consultant Surgeon, The Middlesex Hospital, London, UK

Surgeons need to communicate. The written word is an opportunity to communicate with a wider audience. The prime need for the surgeon is to communicate in a surgical journal about matters of surgical note. Unless a topic has strict application to surgery, it is better written in a non surgical journal. Your colleagues want to read about matters that affect their day to day life.

It is natural that the first stimulus to a young surgeon's writing career is a case report as the apprentice learns and gains experience from individual patients. To be able to present a written or oral case report is the first pre-requisite to a career in surgical communication. With further experience the apprentice has a wider knowledge and is aware that a cohort of patients can be of greater value than the experience of the single interesting presentation.

Writing is for pleasure and for interest. Unless at some stage there is pleasure and interest, writing merely to fulfil a career goal will rarely achieve its objective. As interest in the art of surgery increases so the technical nuance becomes the absorbing factor. Few are granted the privilege of inventing a new operation but the application of a new technology to improve an operation is an exciting experience for the writer.

Any laboratory based research has to be carefully and often laboriously formulated with a relevant hypothesis. Once that formulation has been achieved the process of publishing laboratory work follows naturally. The nearest clinical situation to laboratory based research is the clinical trial and this is correctly emphasised. Those who have participated will be aware that the majority of work occurs before the trial starts and the paper could be written at this stage. Scientific scrutiny is correctly emphasised. This lesson can be used to review subjects, bringing out from a series of relevant articles, messages which have otherwise been missed because of the narrow focus of many authors.

Editorials should be fun to read and fun to write.

Once the disciplines of writing have been mastered the tedium of writing, be it chapters or other communications, will disappear and be replaced by the satisfaction of seeing your work in glossy print; heed the points made in this article and be watchful for opportunities.

Chapter 3

Where can the surgeon publish?

M. Schein

*Professor of Surgery, Cornell University Medical College
& Bronx Lebanon Hospital, New York, U.S.A.*

A. Fingerhut

*Chief of Service, Digestive Surgery, Centre Hospitalier
Intercommunal, Poissy, France & Associate Professor of Surgery
Louisiana State University Medical School
New Orleans, LA, U.S.A.*

Chapter
3

'The unpublished manuscript is like an unconfessed sin that festers in the soul, corrupting and contaminating it' **Antonio Machado**.

In the previous two chapters you were told why [1] and what [2] a surgeon might publish. This chapter will suggest where you can publish whatever publishable material you have. Which target journal is a decision you have to take at the start, before starting to hammer the typewriter keys. When doing the actual writing you have to address the audience you are catering for and keep in mind the specific requirements of the journal you chose. Is your aim to 'sell' a 'new operation' to the general practitioners in your country? In that case you have to emphasize basic concepts. If your purpose is to increase your fame within the surgical community then you can afford to be more technical.

You worked so hard on your study (or so you think) and now you want it to reach the greatest possible and the most prestigious readership, and to have maximal impact. How sweet it could be, strolling around the hospital and repeatedly hearing 'Hey Dr Jones, your *New England Medical Journal* article is superb!' But is your article publishable in such a leading journal? If not, where is it publishable?

Chief goals when looking for a suitable venue for your manuscript

- The greatest readership. Do you wish to bury your *magnum opus* in a 'prestigious' journal that nobody reads?
- An 'interested' readership. You do not want to describe your recent technical innovation to medical gastroenterologists.
- A 'prestigious' journal (high 'impact'). Do not forget - one of the chief reasons for you to publish is the want of prestige [1].
- Maximize chances and speed of acceptance. How depressing it is to submit a 'classic' to a journal that takes a year to reject it.

♦ Minimize rejections and need for prolonged efforts at 'recycling'. Ideally, you want your manuscript to be accepted on the first submission. In reality, a mean of two rejections per manuscript is what you have to live with, unless you are a renowned surgical Shakespeare.

These goals do not always go together. A journal may be 'prestigious-high impact' but attract only a small, narrow-focused readership (e.g. *Journal of Endovascular Surgery*; impact factor (IF) 3.276) or it may have a wide readership, which is, however, not interested in the topic discussed. When 'shopping' for a journal, the manuscript is your merchandise. You have to understand the 'publishing market' and be able to assess the 'value' of your manuscript; only then will it be possible to tailor your manuscript to the individual journal and thus achieve the goals.

The 'market' for the surgical manuscript

Professional journals, as any other commodity, can be graded into 'classes'. The car market has its Rolls Royce, Mercedes, Fords, Toyotas and even Fiats. Which journal is the Jaguar and which the VW Beetle? At this point you should understand the concept of the IF. This is used by the scientific community to score the 'prestige' of individual journals and thus the 'academic value' of the papers published in them. The IF of a journal is calculated as the ratio of the number of citations of articles published by a journal over 2 years (in the whole literature) to the number of articles published over 2 years (by a journal). In simple terms, the more cited the journal, in other publications, the higher its IF. A journal that publishes a relatively small number of novel-momentous papers will have a high IF while a journal accepting a lot of 'non-significant' material is doomed in terms of IF. It is easy to imagine the existence of two separate vicious circles. One involves a high IF journal (e.g. *New England Journal of Medicine*; IF 29.512) which, because of its conceived prestige, attracts the best manuscripts from most qualified investigators and rejects all that is

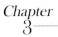

TABLE 1 The market for surgical publishing

ISI Journal Citation Report (Science Edition) 2000

	Impact factor
Class I. 'General top four'. Leading, high-impact and widely read international journals serving all specialties	
New England Journal of Medicine	29.512
JAMA	15.402
Lancet	10.232
British Medical Journal	5.331
Class II. General surgical journals	
IIA. Top group: leading, high-impact and widely read (worldwide) general surgical journals	
Annals of Surgery	5.987
British Journal of Surgery	2.935
Journal of the American College of Surgeons	2.805
Annals of Surgical Oncology	2.799
Archives of Surgery	2.629
Surgery	2.456
American Journal of Surgery	2.116
World Journal of Surgery	2.020
Arch Langenbeck Surgery (German)	1.770
Journal of Surgical Research	1.674
Journal of Surgical Oncology	1.541
European Journal of Surgical Oncology	1.434
American Surgeon	1.101
IIB. Intermediate group	
Hepatogastroenterology	0.905
Digestive Surgery	0.810
Der Chirurg (German)	0.721
European Journal of Surgery	0.663
Australian and New Zealand Journal of Surgery	0.627
Annales de Chirurgie (French)	0.545
Journal of the Royal College of Surgeons of Edinburgh	0.510
International Surgery	0.488
Annals of the Royal College of Surgeons of England	0.439
Canadian Journal of Surgery	0.422
Surgery Today	0.356
Zentralblatt Chirurgie (German)	0.302

TABLE 1 *continued*
The market for surgical publishing

	Impact factor
IIC. 'Bottom' group	
Surgical Oncology	0.293
Minimally Invasive Therapy	0.291
Acta Chirurgica Belgica (French)	0.270
Journal de Chirurgie (Paris) (French)	0.213
South African Journal of Surgery	0.159
Contemporary Surgery	--*
Current Surgery	--*
Surgical Rounds	--*
Journal of Surgical Infections	--*
Class III. Subspecialty journals	
IIIA. Top group: leading, high-impact and widely read (worldwide) subspecialty surgical and 'surgical interest' journals	
Gastroenterology	12.246
Transplantation	4.035
Critical Care Medicine	3.824
Cancer	3.611
Journal of Endovascular Surgery	3.276
Journal of Vascular Surgery	3.114
Journal of Thoracic and Cardiovascular Surgery	3.057
Shock	2.785
Surgical Endoscopy and Ultrasonography	2.056
IIIB. Lower group	
Annals of Thoracic Surgery	1.828
Diseases of the Colon and Rectum	1.690
Journal of Trauma	1.498
Obesity Surgery	1.464
Journal of Pediatric Surgery	1.216
Journal of Laparoendoscopic Surgery	0.783
Surgical Laparoscopy and Endoscopy	0.691
Vascular Surgery	0.627**

Class IV. 'Local' journals: general or specialty journals published in your country, usually in your language

* New journals, not as yet cited by the Journal Citation report. The list of journals is not inclusive. A grading of journals using the impact factor is prone to bias as explained in the text. To access the web page on any of the listed journals go to: Land of Medical Links by Joe Buenker: http://alexia.lis.uiuc.edu/~buenker/journla.html

** ISI Journal Citation Report (Science Edition) 1998

inferior. Its publications are 'best-sellers' and highly quoted across the world, thus further increasing the IF. On the other hand, a 'modest' journal such as the *European Journal of Surgery* starts with a much lower IF (0.663) and consequently attracts manuscripts of 'lesser value', and may be forced to publish papers rejected by others. The latter are poorly cited thus the journal's IF remains low. While it is very difficult to improve a journal's IF, it is very easy to lose it by poor editorial performance. The IF as a gauging instrument is far from perfect: it favours English-language, 'large specialties', the USA and journals with fewer articles. It hinders predominantly clinical journals. Table 1 shows the IF of different journals classified into a number of groups, based on the IF and a personal perception of the surgical 'publishing market'.

Whether the IF has any impact on readers has hitherto received very little attention. In a Chinese study of library journal use there was a significant correlation between frequency of use and IF [3]. An assessment of journals used at a Chicago medical library found that certain journals may be popular to the general reader, for educational and clinical purposes, but not to the local faculty for research purposes [4]. In a recent survey on what American surgeons read [5], it was found that IF correlates only partially with the 'importance' attributed to the various journals by surgeons. Other factors were important; for example, certain journals are 'forced' on surgeons as part of a membership package of large surgical associations.

What is the value of your manuscript?

To most writers, especially the novice, a recently completed study seems a potential masterpiece, which deserves the best venue and audience. (Only last week one of our residents in New York suggested that his humble series of three 'unusual' cases should be written up for the *Lancet*.) To maximize the chances of acceptance of your alleged 'masterwork' you have to assess its quality. This should provide a realistic view of the value of the paper and direct you to the right journal. For example, a retrospective clinical series is not going to get published in the *New England Journal of Medicine*. In Table 2 a practical classification of 'original studies' is proposed. The latter, however, should not be lumped together with 'review articles' or 'technical notes' but the value of each should be assessed within its own kind.

TABLE 2
What is the 'value' of your manuscript?

Level	Description	Example	Submit to
I	Groundbreaking discovery, high level of evidence; if reconfirmed may radically change clinical practice	'A new operation for anal incontinence - 5 years' follow-up in 500 patients' or 'Laparoscopic versus conventional Whipple procedure: a prospective randomized trial in 200 patients'	Class I or IIA journals (see Table 1)
II	Novel and/or well performed piece of research that may significantly change current thinking or modify (or enhance) clinical practice	'Gene transfer therapy of hepatic cancer' or 'Conservative versus operative treatment of recurrent acute diverticulitis: a prospective randomized study with a 3-year follow-up' or 'The value of preoperative bowel preparation - a meta-analysis'	Class IIA or IIIA journals (see Table 1)
III	A solid piece of research that sheds new light or confirms/ disputes what is already known	'Faecal diversion is not necessary in low anterior resection of the rectum - experience in 99 patients'	Class IIA, IIB, IIIA or IIIB journals (see Table 1)
IV	A 'nice little study'; local experience with a known entity or a 'reminder' about a rare condition	'Upper gastrointestinal bleeding in Scandinavia' or 'Acute appendicitis after appendicectomy - report of five cases'	Class IIC or IV journals (see Table 1)

How to select the right journal for your manuscript

When you know how to assess the prestige of the various journals and can estimate objectively the worth of your work, how easy is it to correctly match the two together? It is difficult and requires experience but the following is a practical advice list.

♦ Choose the audience - general, specialized or local? If you have data for a level II paper (Table 2) on surgical gastroenterology, you may aim for the top of class IIA journals (Table 1), reaching the cream of surgical readership. Alternatively you could select a leading class IIIA subspecialty journal (Table 1) in gastroenterology, targeting mainly those interested in this field, surgeons and non-surgeons.

- ◆ Consult the 'instructions to authors'. These are available in each journal. See what type of manuscript they prefer. Read the aims and objectives or mission statement of the journal. All journals welcome 'original' clinical and laboratory studies but only some consider review articles, pure technical notes or case reports. Only a few accept non-commissioned editorials. Studying the instructions to authors is a *sine qua non*. Submitting an unsuitable manuscript results in an automatic rejection. At this stage you may short list a few journals for an in-depth analysis.

- ◆ Browse through the journals. See what type of papers they published over the past year. Would your manuscript fit the ethos and style of that journal?

- ◆ If the journal has already published one or two articles on 'your topic', you might want to go elsewhere. If your paper can solve the problem raised by a previous article in that journal, go ahead.

- ◆ Some surgeons make a habit of submitting all their papers to one journal or a limited list of journals. This may not be a bad idea as they gradually learn how to satisfy the needs of these journals while the latter become familiar with them.

- ◆ Get advice. Choosing a journal for your manuscript is an art that is acquired during many years of submission-rejection, trial-error cycles. As editorial reviewers for a number of journals, we often see manuscripts that are misdirected into the 'wrong' journal. This represents a waste of efforts by the authors, reviewers and journal editors, which could be avoided if the author first consults an experienced and well published surgeon in their environment. A well published and well read surgeon has a 'publishing judgement' which, like clinical judgement, is difficult to express in any algorithm. His skills allow him to penetrate into the mind of the various journal editors and reviewers, guessing what they like and what they dislike. He knows which journals are 'rigid-traditional' and which would consider 'innovative' styles. He knows the assessment-rejection cycle of the individual journals and can advise you how high to start and how to continue, maximizing the rate of eventual acceptance and its speed. If no such an expert is available in your vicinity try elsewhere; no surgeon would refuse to give advice to a young colleague. Journal editors themselves may give you an informal view of a proposed article.

Getting your paper published is a complex task, which is becoming increasingly difficult. Only a few decades ago prestigious journals published long manuscripts based on three clinical cases; now you cannot publish the most interesting case reports outside local or 'throw-away' journals. Rejection rates are extremely high, e.g. 80 per cent for the *BJS*. A key element of a successful submission is choosing the right journal. Assess the value of your manuscript, know the publishing market, study the target journals and get learned advice.

Acknowledgements

The authors thank Dr Asher Hirshberg for advice and Dr Ramesh Paladugu for helping with the data and tables.

References

1   Schein M, Farndon JR, Fingerhut A. Why should a surgeon publish? *Br J Surg* 2000; 87: 3-5.

2   O'Connell PR. What should surgeons write? *Br J Surg* 2000; 87: 132-4.

3   Tsay MY. The relationship between journal use in a medical library and citation use. *Bull Med Libr Assoc* 1998; 86: 31-9.

4   Blecic DD. Measurements of journal use: an analysis of the correlations between three methods. *Bull Med Libr Assoc* 1999; 871: 20-5.

5   Schein M, Paladugu R, Sutija V, Wise L. What American Surgeons Read: a survey of a thousand Fellows of the American College of Surgeons. *Curr Surg* 2000; 57: 252-258.

Commentary
by J. L. Meakins
Archibald Professor of Surgery, McGill University
Montreal, Canada

The opening quote suggests that everything that we study and write up is worth publishing. While it is certainly true - IF IT IS NOT PUBLISHED, IT DOES NOT EXIST - our ability to evaluate our own work and to determine its publication value is not only an important part of selecting the appropriate journal but also deciding whether it should see the light of day. I have drawers full of material which at one time seemed to be priceless insights into the understanding of the infectious process, a clinical entity or the integration of a bench observation and a pathophysiologic process. Before asking the question 'Where should I publish?', we must be certain that what is in the drawer is actually publishable. Then ask, 'is it publishable in its present form?'.

I do not think that I have ever submitted an article with any thought being given to the Impact Factor of the journal. Writers should be readers. By reading the literature, one gets a sense not only of what is out there but also where work should be published. This nose for the right journal is emphasised in the point - GET ADVICE. In the spirit that we should read more of the literature than we write, this nose will come naturally and rather quickly if the quality of the insights brought to research is applied to journals. One does get more points in the promotion game with few papers in the very high impact journals. However, a reality check will demonstrate that not very many publish often in these journals and that most of us do not very often produce work that is sufficiently meritorious to do so.

One of the useful methods of deciding where to publish can be related to where the work is presented. Many associations and societies have their own journals or arrangements with journals to review manuscripts submitted for presentation. In this way the research is presented before a knowledgeable audience and has a good chance of being published as part of the transactions of the meeting.

Increasingly, journals are less interested in some of the classic surgical papers such as chart reviews, personal series, case reports, minimal publishable units (20 rats in 4 groups of 5 or 2 groups of 10), retrospective uncontrolled studies or clinical studies with the wrong or no control groups. The best solution is not to do these studies and therefore avoid the angst of rejection. Don't send bench research to a clinical journal or vice-versa. You will receive a rejection and a poor assessment from the review process.

When our assessment of our work includes words such as 'Magnum opus', 'classic', and 'want of prestige', it is possible that one is losing track of why the work was done in the first place. Scholarship is the fundamental drive behind the development of new information, which surely is the reason that we publish in the first place. Our *ability to assess the work is therefore crucial. The observation that 'a mean of two rejections per manuscript' is usual, I find hardly credible. One rejection with careful attention to the comments of the referees should be sufficient to define whether the material is publishable and where the author is most likely to be successful. It is not the amount of effort that goes into the manuscript but its quality that is important. Quality refers not only to the content but also to the quality of the writing. One of the most important lessons I learned was from a very short letter from the Editor of The Lancet: 'If you could bear to shorten your paper by a third, we would be happy to publish'.*

Chapter 4

*Generating
an idea: will it
be publishable?*

M. G. Sarr

Professor of Surgery

Mayo Clinic

Rochester, Minnesota, U.S.A.

While ideas are plentiful and often appear to the originator as novel, interesting, and exciting, the actual formulation of this idea into a final product of interest to an editor and to the journal's readership often represents the more difficult part. Many young aspiring surgical authors are (understandably) naïve about the entire process of idea development, background research (there is always much more written about a topic than the budding author ever imagined), packaging this idea into a worthy manuscript, and finally the appropriate process of submission/review/acceptance. Many young authors do not appreciate that just as the practice of surgery requires education and training, medical writing and publication also requires a formal training which involves research, advice from peers and mentors/teachers, and just plain hard work. While editors of journals are eager to publish good work and will actively encourage promising ideas, it is incumbent on the authors to write an appropriate, complete manuscript. Ideas are not publishable - manuscripts are!

While this introduction seems pessimistic to starting a career in publishing (or for that matter in getting any idea published), it should not be taken so. Writing is fun, especially when you have been able to nurture and grow an idea that ends up on paper (or these days in the electronic medium) in a nicely packaged, cogent, convincing form. It is even more fun for many authors when the manuscript comes out in the journal or book as a finished, published piece. In this respect, prospective authors should be encouraged and not discouraged to pursue their ideas and to write them up BUT only after obtaining advice and help from someone with experience in medical publishing.

This chapter is designed to provide guidelines to young or more naïve authors in an attempt to help focus development of ideas into a publishable article. The ideas in this chapter represent primarily my personal views on concept of both publishing and idea-development. These ideas are based not only on my experience as an author but on more recent experience as a co-editor of the journal *Surgery*.

This chapter will concentrate on generating a publishable idea based on the various types of submissions (Table 1). I provide key concepts for the prospective author to consider before embarking on work into a topic or approach that is, predictably, doomed from the start. Prior to addressing each type of submission, several overall concepts (Table 2) should be of help.

♦ Run your 'idea' past someone with experience in medical publishing before you begin.

♦ Ask for help in organizing, researching, analyzing, and writing up the idea.

♦ Listen to the advice and constructive criticism given.

♦ Make the title and topic 'sexy;' you want the editor and the reader to want to read it!

♦ Before submitting your 'final' manuscript, have someone with experience read and criticize it - be prepared both to accept constructive criticism and to change the manuscript.

♦ Keep your idealism, but be realistic.

♦ Some ideas are not publishable.

♦ Start out with a 'single' rather than trying to hit a 'home run.'

Types of submissions

Case Report

While case reports are usually quite focused and often may be a nice and convenient, easy way to start out in medical publishing, these types of reports are all-too-often difficult to justify and may be very

35

TABLE 1
Available Formats of Publication*

Type of format	Key concepts
Case report	Unique, novel, educational, broad-interest, practical
Technique paper	New, innovative, well-illustrated, outcome-based clinical experience helps
Cohort study and case series	Focused problem, adequate number of patients, appropriate follow-up, objective outcome measures, aim/hypothesis.
Case-controlled studies	Insight into factors affecting outcomes, non-biased care selection of case controls
Prospective study	Plan well before beginning
Non-randomized	Established practice or well-accepted controls
Randomized	Adequate power, statistical validity, single or double blinded
Review article	Broad interest, education, controversy, recent consensus
Meta-analysis	Methodology and evaluable published studies are crucial, a statistician is imperative
Editorial	Usually invited, not as free submissions, written by recognized authorities
Letter-to-the-editor	Justified constructive (not destructive) criticism, broad interest, non-parochial
Images section	Spectacular, clear visual image, unusual clinical case with visual picture
Research paper	Hypothesis-driven, mechanistic (vs phenomenological), clinical or basic, especially translational, state-of-the-art technology, scientifically valid

Adapted from Sarr (2000)[1]

hard or impossible to get published. Many of the current journals are shying away from publishing case reports - especially the case reports addressing the extremely unusual or rare condition. While interesting from a theoretical standpoint or because this problem 'may never have been reported before,' if the case report does nothing more than catalogue the phenomenon, most journals will not be interested. Editors look for new or novel problems that offer insight into disease processes, provide novel approaches to treatment, or provide broad educational benefit.

Avoid falling prey to the erroneous belief that just because it is the 'first' report of this condition, it warrants publication. Be extremely careful to claim that your report is the 'first reported case;' the literature goes back well over 100 years, and you had better have done a very careful and complete review of the literature - not just a computer search of several key words. Authors of previous publications about the same topic will be quite anxious to point out your oversight in a rapidly submitted (and embarrassing) letter to the editor. Although a 'weird neoplasm,' a 'really fascinating presentation,' an 'unusual complication,' or a problem 'I've never seen before' may indeed intrigue you and your colleagues, such a topic is not always of sufficient interest for publication unless it offers useful information for the readership. A case report should be novel, unique, or timely. It should be of broad-enough interest to capture a sizeable segment of that journal's readership. Those case reports that provide a lesson that is practical, novel and educational are the most attractive.

Finally, be selective in the journal to which you send your case report. Some journals NEVER publish case reports - do not waste your time with those journals - your fascinating case will not change their policy. If your case is very organ-, topic- or specialty-specific, select a focused subspecialty journal, not a broad-based surgical journal that has a very broad readership.

TABLE 2

General Advice

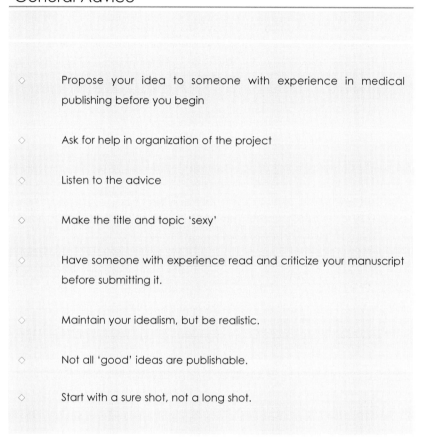

◇   Propose your idea to someone with experience in medical publishing before you begin

◇   Ask for help in organization of the project

◇   Listen to the advice

◇   Make the title and topic 'sexy'

◇   Have someone with experience read and criticize your manuscript before submitting it.

◇   Maintain your idealism, but be realistic.

◇   Not all 'good' ideas are publishable.

◇   Start with a sure shot, not a long shot.

Technique Paper

Technique papers should clearly describe the operative technique of interest and should include figures to illustrate certain key points. A publishable technique paper should offer some technical aspect that is novel or innovative. Writing up a manuscript describing 'the Master's technique' at University X for performing a specific procedure may not of itself be of sufficient interest for a journal to devote a few pages. Remember two things: first, there are many 'masters' in many university and non-university centres, all of which have their own 'special techniques'. Second, new techniques are rare and were often learned from others (thus not new) or adapted from other procedures (and thus not always novel). Beware the concept of idolatry of 'the master' - while often appropriate in your parochial environment, if you have not visited other centres and observed how other masters carry out the same operation, don't necessarily be naïve enough to think that no one else has the insight to have figured out the same or similar novel 'new' techniques.

Several caveats should be mentioned. Good, clear, professional (not hand-drawn) illustrations are usually mandatory. Be simple but clear. On occasion, very detailed drawings are necessary, but often such detail detracts from the basic technique you wish to portray. Make the figures appropriate but as simple as possible. Limit the number of figures used; it will be very hard to justify a de novo, unsolicited technique paper with three to five figures. Finally, adequate clinical experience to justify the outcome of the technique is imperative; description of a new technique in just one patient will not arouse much interest. A new or novel technique that is safe and effective, as justified by an objectively defined clinical experience of several patients with a defined patient outcome, will be looked on much more favourably by the journal.

Several exceptions are pertinent. On occasion, a general description of the operative technique of a truly internationally renowned surgeon may be of interest even if the technique is not especially novel. Similarly, on occasion certain journals will have a section on 'How I do it' consisting of an invited manuscript on a technique by an expert in the field. These, however, are the exceptions.

Cohort Study and Case Series

These types of publications probably represent the largest category of clinically oriented surgical literature. The concept behind these reports rests on reporting an experience of treating a group of patients with the same disease process. Usually, these reports are retrospective, chart-type reviews of patient presentations, techniques of diagnosis, and/or outcomes after either a uniform treatment or after several different treatments in an attempt to compare one's experience with that reported in the literature.

Good, solid cohort studies or case series depend on a focused, well-defined problem or disease process. To provide useful data on presentation, diagnosis, outcome, etc., it is incumbent on the author to have adequate numbers of patients, measurable outcome criteria (morbidity, mortality, quality-of-life), and a satisfactory, reasonably complete follow-up of long enough duration. For instance, follow-up of less than 2 years would be unsatisfactory for a manuscript on hernia repair. Reliance on the justification for publication being the series comes from your 'world famous' institution will not be satisfactory by itself.

When preparing a case series or cohort study, several suggestions can help in the planning and preparation of the manuscript. Inclusion of an aim of the work and a reasonable hypothesis based on previous literature markedly strengthens the work. Similarly, the topic addressed should be relevant to the journal's readership and of sufficient surgical interest. A simple catalogue of your institutional experience with operative treatment of disease X does not always justify publication. These types of manuscripts are much more attractive if the diagnosis or treatment described offers a new approach or unique analysis not previously defined. Interestingly, sometimes a very poor outcome may itself justify publication. This author believes strongly that it might even be incumbent on authors to report poor outcomes of ostensibly 'accepted' or 'new' procedures so that others do not perpetuate bad clinical approaches.

Case Control Series

These manuscripts compare a select group of patients, for instance, undergoing a certain treatment or operation with an ostensibly random group of age, sex, or other form of 'matched' patients undergoing the same treatment. This form of comparison is stronger than cohort or case series comparing two groups of patients matched only for method of treatment. Obviously, the case control approach is only as good as the method of choosing controls. This type of approach is most appropriate for a group of patients in whom marked differences in age, comorbidities, or gender might be expected to alter outcomes. This type of publication, while much more reliable, implies some insight into factors affecting outcome and requires utilization of a non-biased, careful selection of case controls.

Prospective Studies

These studies are currently accepted as the most powerful type of clinical research study and represent the gold standard. For a young or aspiring surgeon, these studies require considerable forethought and preparation because they usually take several years (or decades) to mature and acquire enough clinical material for meaningful analysis - especially for the more rare, unusual disorders. Thus, the surgeon must be able to be patient and will only begin to reap the benefits (i.e. publication[s]) after the clinical work has been completed. This approach usually requires a permanent job at an institution without aspirations of moving to another location and a dedication and perseverance to pursue the original idea. Retrospective studies report on clinical outcomes of work done by you or others and in essence involve an analysis of what has already been done, while prospective studies assume a planned design to evaluate some preconceived aim and hypothesis. This approach assumes insight into important questions able to be constructed and answered by the study.

The strengths of prospective studies lie in the primary assumption of hypothesis-driven work. A problem or question is formulated, a plan developed, and then the study begins with prospective collection of data. This approach represents a very strong methodology that should obviate the shortcomings of a retrospective study, i.e. hindsight and inability to evaluate or assess certain important parameters. A prospective study is only as good as the study design and the type, methodology, and completeness of data collection. Because prospective studies may take years to complete, the aspiring author must be able to wait for maturation before the study is publishable. If the person developing and organizing the study will not be at that institution for the duration of study, the personal benefit of the study for that individual may be largely lost, and thus the concept of 'What's in it for me?' Authorship may still be agreed even though participation is only in the development phase.

- *Prospective non-randomized study*

This approach is commonly used to develop databases of focused disorders, diseases or operations assuming a specific treatment. The prospective collection of data represents the major strength. However, if there is no formal or statistical comparison to another group of patients (see below, Randomized prospective studies), much of the potential strength of a prospective study is lost. A large database can be used to write manuscripts on multiple aspects of the problem of interest. These types of studies are most effective when you plan to compare your treatment approach with other well-described or accepted approaches for which outcome data are available. Otherwise these studies become 'this is what we did and here are our results' and without a comparison group these results are less meaningful.

Several considerations prior to beginning such a study are important. The data to be collected represents the meat of the future work. Considerable forethought should be given to be certain the database is exhaustive. Get advice from someone who has developed a database. Talk to a computer programmer about organization, methods of collection, data entry, and internal checks within the database in an attempt to recognize input errors as the data are entered. There is little worse in a prospective study than having to clean the database of multiple clerical errors of data input. The final product is only as good as the accuracy of the data entered. All too often the importance of a crucial variable which was not evaluated during the study is only recognized at the end of the study. This defeats the entire purpose of the prospective nature of the study.

Special effort should be devoted to quantification of variables. For instance, subjective evaluations are much more difficult to quantitate (e.g. pain, quality of life) than are direct variables (age, sex, and laboratory values). Validated methodologies and expertise in using these methodologies exists, but they must be determined before starting the study. It is better to develop a planned data collection protocol and have it reviewed by several local experts before starting the study. If crucial variables are not collected prospectively, the advantages of a prospective study are lost. Considerable time spent planning the study before starting is well worth it when analyzing the results and writing the manuscript later.

◆ *Prospective, randomized study*

For clinical questions that are testable, this format represents the gold standard. These studies can be single-blinded (the patient does not know which treatment he/she received) or double-blinded (neither patient nor physician knows). Some forms of therapy cannot be either blinded (operation vs no operation) or double-blinded (one form of therapy requires that the physician knows the treatment administered). In these situations, every attempt at avoiding reviewer or analyst bias must be assured to maintain appropriate randomization and collection/analysis of data. As with non-randomized prospective studies, the design and planning of the study before it begins is crucial.

First, the study must be adequately powered with enough patients to statistically answer the question. This assumes that the investigator has a reasonable guess or idea of the rate of expected outcomes and can identify a 'success' that will be considered 'clinically important.' For instance, treatment X has a 20% complication rate; treatment Y would be accepted as a better treatment if the complication rate can be decreased to 10%; i.e. 50% reduction in complications. Using a power calculation (here is where a statistician is imperative), one can then determine the minimum number of patients per treatment group to provide a result that reaches statistical significance. There is nothing worse than an underpowered study with too few patients and, although nicely done and completed, if there are too few patients, no conclusions can be reached.

Second - try to avoid post hoc analyses. These analyses are done after the study has been completed and are attempts to compare subgroups or treatments that were not part of the original power analysis. These analyses are often based on observations made during the study of what appear to the investigator to be 'trends.' While sometimes important and meaningful, post hoc analyses are usually strongly challenged and questioned. They are usually 'after the fact' analyses done because the study seemed to suggest an effect. Remember the study was not designed to address this question and a post hoc analysis is a form of retrospective analysis and often there are too few patients to confidently answer the question.

Finally, be prepared for a very careful, comprehensive review by your institutional human studies review board. If you have not carefully read all the criteria needed for such a prospective, randomized study (consent form, funding, interim analysis, adverse events, serious adverse events, etc.), then you are not ready to submit your proposed protocol. Be prepared for it to take time for the study to be evaluated and approved (usually 1-2 months minimum).

Review Article

In the past, this type of a publication served as a possible avenue for young or inexperienced surgeons without personal experience. However many journals are no longer accepting review submissions that are not 'invited.' Thus, before embarking on a time-consuming, laborious library research, be certain that there is a journal appropriate and receptive to such an article.

Several concepts about review articles should be considered before starting. Review articles can serve several purposes. Usually, these articles address topics of broad interest that provide considerable educational benefit, provided sufficient data exists to provide that educational benefit. Other possible concepts that might support the usefulness of such a review article are whether the planned review will fill a sufficient gap in current understanding either in common clinical practice, recent textbooks, or recent literature. Other potentially important questions are the following: Will the review capture the interest of the editor (as well as the readership)? Are there any ongoing unanswered controversies you can further discuss and/or clarify? Has a consensus been reached recently that is not well known? Will the article be too focused? Will the review article be of only unsophisticated educational interest? The prospective author should remember that most state-of-the-art journals or the high-visibility journals with the highest citation index will not be interested in a purely pedestrian educational review.

If the decision to pursue a review article is made, be careful to review all the literature. Several search engines and key words should be used, not just a Medline search. All articles quoted should be found and read by the author rather than taking references from other articles. It is disappointing to see how 'classic' papers are either misquoted or mis-referenced and then these misquotes and incorrect references are perpetuated in subsequent literature because the original article was not read and/or the reference was not checked for accuracy. Similarly, an attempt at reviewing articles in other languages should be made, or at the least, you should be careful to acknowledge that only the English language literature was reviewed. Be very careful if you claim an article (or author) to be the first report.

Meta-analyses

Meta-analyses attempt to address a question by combining the results of many previous studies into a common analysis to obtain a statistically appropriate and valid number or sample of patients or episodes of treatment to answer a question. This type of analysis requires an adequate number of published studies that fulfil criteria for inclusion concerning such concepts as appropriate categories of patients, clearly definable and objective measures of outcome, and adequate follow-up. Thus, for a meta-analysis to be sound and justified, its methodology must be valid. This latter group of concepts is critical because not all questions of interest are amenable to a meta-analysis.

Currently, most journals are very careful about accepting meta-analyses for publication. Appropriate meta-analyses require close cooperation and collaboration with an experienced statistician in the design, data retrieval, and analysis to be used. This collaboration should be sought before designing the study or beginning the analysis. Most physicians and surgeons are not trained or versed in the statistical methods required of a good, valid meta-analysis. In addition, a careful, thorough, comprehensive, and critical review of the literature is imperative. A good meta-analysis can only be as good as the literature on which it is based. Publication bias must be controlled for, in that most journals prefer to publish a study with a positive outcome rather than one where there is no difference or an adverse outcome from a new technique or treatment.

Editorial

Editorials are virtually always written by either the editor(s) of the journal or by a recognized expert in the field invited to do so by the journal. Do not confuse letters to the editor with editorials. Unsolicited editorials to journals are usually not well accepted, especially from the naïve, aspiring author. Your critique of an article is better addressed as a brief, focused letter to the editor (see below) rather than an attempt to have the journal publish your views as an editorial. While everyone is entitled to an opinion, convincing a journal to devote a precious page for your opinion may be next to impossible.

Letter to the Editor

This 'publication' serves as a potential sounding board for criticism of past articles published in that journal or for additional personal support of recent articles. General rules of thumb might be the following: keep the letter short and to the point; avoid solely your own parochial interests; make the letter more one of constructive rather than destructive criticism; and identify potential errors of interpretation; and be certain to justify your critique. Remember - if accepted, the author will have a chance to rebut your letter, so be prepared to accept the response. On occasion, a letter to the editor may report a case (patient) that highlights or further exemplifies or contrasts with a previous article in that journal. Another potential topic might be a 'mini-study' you have conducted that by itself will not stand as a full manuscript.

Images Section

Recently, several surgical journals have adopted a short, usually 1-page section. Examples include an educational radiograph, a photograph of a patient or clinical findings, histopathology or gross pathology, or visual examples of special research interest (e.g. Northern or Western blot, immunofluorescence, etc.). Some of these images are common disorders that clearly demonstrate a clinical scenario (e.g. pneumobilia in a patient with a small bowel obstruction from an impacted gallstone) or may represent an avenue for reporting an interesting but rare or previously unreported clinical experience. The published images (usually no more than 2 or 3) are rather spectacular and dramatic and serve to clearly demonstrate an often pathognomonic visual picture. Some images sections have a short discussion of the clinical setting, while others will have a one or two paragraph overview of the topic as a whole. These clinicopathological correlations are meant to be short and educational, not the basis for an exhaustive review of the literature.

Basic Research Paper

Ironically, these types of submissions may actually be easier to publish in a more clinically oriented journal than the true clinical studies, probably because the impression by many naïve authors, or even some editors, is that bench research papers have more inherent credence (and worth) than clinical papers. This common misconception is even more true when techniques of molecular biology are included in the manuscript (e.g. Northern blots, Western blots, gel shifts, etc.). However, good science is good science, and bad science is bad science wherever it is published.

Before embarking on a bench research study, first be careful to do your 'research' about the lab you are planning to join - mentor, technicians, post-docs, facilities and opportunities. Probably most important, talk with your colleagues, fellows, medical students, or other post docs who have worked in the lab before you. They often (usually) provide the best advice. Second, your research 'idea' which you plan to pursue needs to be well thought out. What may sound very unique, novel, and new to you may very likely have been done, might not be practical, or might be of very little interest to experts or importance in the field. Third, remember that you are just starting; there is always far more literature on a topic than you ever thought possible. Finally, when first starting out, set your sights low. Tackle a problem that is straightforward, able to be finished, and is attainable. Rather than taking up a long shot, pick a sure shot even if it may not be as dramatic. Try for a 'single,' rather than a 'home run.' You want your first project to be successful. Success breeds further success. Once you have become established, then the risky gambles can be tried; if unsuccessful, the loss is not as great.

Summary

The above advice is offered in an attempt to encourage young surgeons to pursue academic work that will be published. Not only is academia fun and exciting, it is also very rewarding, especially when your published work makes a durable contribution. Hopefully the above discussion will provide overall guidelines and criteria for the naïve author; there is nothing worse to the aspiring author than to receive a negative review, especially if it was predictable or preventable with some forethought and helpful advice. Many submissions are doomed from the start because of flaws in design, analysis, data collection, or submission to inappropriate journals.

The best possible advice to the young, new, or beginning author is to seek the help and advice of a seasoned veteran. While it may be best to begin to plan the project, do some preliminary research, and formulate an approach prior to seeking advice, the insightful aspiring author should not commit too much time and effort into collecting and analyzing data and writing a potential manuscript for potential submission before getting the constructive advice from an expert. Good ideas that are well developed, well planned, and complete are published, but bad ideas or poorly designed and planned ideas are rejected.

References

1   Sarr MG. Generating an idea: will it be publishable? *Br J Surg* 2000; 87: 388-389.

Commentary
by N. O'Higgins

**Senior Professor of Surgery, University College Dublin,
St. Vincent's University Hospital, Dublin, Ireland**

The title of the chapter suggests that 'ideas in surgery' might be publishable. It raises the interesting question as to what type of journal in the surgical arena would accept evidence-based hypotheses or ideas which might stimulate research activity. Insufficient space in surgical journals is devoted to publishing 'ideas' or surgical concepts which might be testable. This chapter deals almost exclusively with the different types of publication possible rather than how ideas might be presented for publication.

Dr. Sarr neatly clarifies the types of papers suitable for submission to medical journals, drawing particular attention to the pitfalls and difficulties involved in preparing each type of publication. He also provides solid and specific advice to authors about the mechanisms of preparing a document in suitable form to make it attractive to editors and readers. Little emphasis is placed on the fundamental need for intensive study of the existing literature on any topic before a paper, whether a case report or basic research paper, is planned and written. Dr. Sarr indicates that writing a paper represents much hard work and perhaps this point can be presumed. All the advice given is pragmatic, sensible and 'smart' even if at times over-simplistic. Is it necessary to advise authors not to send case reports to journals which never publish case reports? Is it necessary to tell young surgeons that there is a distinction between Editorials and Letters-to-the-Editor? It would also have been of interest to read the author's view about how a higher degree in surgery by thesis might be formulated, planned, designed and put together.

This chapter will be useful to all young surgeons in their approach to writing a scientific paper.

Chapter
4

Chapter 5

On getting started

D. Alderson

Professor of Surgery

Bristol Royal Infirmary

Bristol, UK

At some point, the fruits of your research labours must be turned into a final product, which will be read by a critical audience of potentially unlimited size.

Getting Organised

'Annihilate but space and time' **Alexander Pope**

To get a flow of words started, you must collect and organise materials and create an environment free from interruptions. Nobody has produced a useful paper during the breaks in an operating list, no matter how slow the anaesthetist!

The correct environment for reading and writing involves a combination of the right time and place. The task of collating the resources you require in an appropriate environment is an important one and there are key issues to be addressed at this stage. The most important is time. First thing in the morning, late at night, blocks of time each day or weekends will suit individuals differently but the creation of 'new time' to complete this task is highly desirable. You may have completed some other assignment which frees up this time. In general, most people are suited by dividing up work time into short blocks involving different tasks and this tends to increase efficiency.

A few self-imposed deadlines for completion of individual elements of the work is a useful discipline. Whether you prefer to write, type or dictate is a matter of personal preference. The spoken word may help to overcome the problem of 'writer's block' (see below) but it is important to remember that written and spoken languages are different and dictation for a written piece does not come easily to everyone. You will probably find the consequence is that more editorial work will be required. The ability to rapidly 'cut and paste' with modern word-processing makes direct work onto the computer screen attractive to many.

Having decided on the right time, your next task is to find the right place. You may be able to produce the entire paper electronically, but most of us still like to scribble down occasional flashes of inspiration, which just happen to leap into the thought processes at sometimes inconvenient moments. It is worthwhile having a thesaurus or dictionary to hand, particularly for the phases when you rewrite and edit individual sections.

Ensure that your chosen environment will be comfortable, free from distractions and interruptions. A lap top computer during a train or aeroplane journey may be your choice. It is probably the knowledge that there is a defined amount of time in a protected place that makes this so attractive.

While some individuals may find it is helpful to ritually organise their working environment, prolonged desk clearing is really just an act of procrastination appeasing an ill prepared mind. An empty piece of floor is just as useful as a storage space.

Having set time aside and identified your working environment, you now need to gather together all of the reading matter (original scientific articles, published abstracts, review articles and text books) that you will need, along with materials concerned with the investigations you intend to report (grant applications, ethical submissions and study data). Whether you do this electronically or with paper is unimportant. It is vital, however, that the literature search should be exhaustive. Electronic searches of MEDLINE and EMBASE are good starting points. Other electronic resources worth searching include the Cochrane Library, SCISEARCH and BIDS. It is worthwhile at this stage investigating the resources available within your postgraduate or university library, where professional on-line searchers and medical reference librarians may be able to help with a search strategy. MEDLINE goes back only to 1966. A library is still probably the easiest way to access most standard text books and obtain historical papers if they are relevant.

Under no circumstances should you cheat by relying on the reading of abstracts alone or the citation of secondary sources (i.e. theft from the bibliography of another paper). This only compounds errors and perpetuates surgical mythology.

Never forget the more historical literature. There is very little in medicine that is genuinely brand new and it is important to place your work in its own historical context.

Taming the Literature

'There is first the literature of knowledge and secondly,
the literature of power' **Thomas De Quincey**

Hopefully most of your reading was completed before you embarked on the project. In the light of your own research efforts, now is the time for a critical appraisal of this literature. Read, highlight and re-read. Make lists of important points in the format of your choice. Acquire additional references as a result and continue this process until you are certain that the bibliography upon which you intend to rely, is exhaustive. You must learn to be critical and avoid the temptation to be selective or dismissive of material which contradicts your hypothesis or results. The use of a selective bibliography to reinforce a theory, will nearly always lead to rejection by journal referees, if not major criticisms from your co-authors.

The development of this critical faculty is vital, not only for the process of writing but also in starting the entire research process. Its importance cannot be over-emphasised. An easy way to carry out a thorough appraisal of a publication, is to ask six simple questions; why, how, who, what, how many and so what?

<u>Why did the authors do the study?</u> Is the hypothesis clearly stated? If the study involves some sort of therapeutic intervention, is it about efficacy or effectiveness? Efficacy is about a specific outcome under ideal circumstance, whereas effectiveness seeks to determine whether

an intervention does more good than harm in patients under normal clinical circumstances. Consider laparoscopic exploration of the common bile duct as a treatment for choledocholithiasis. To study efficacy, the treatment group will consist of patients with clearly documented stones in the bile duct, all of whom undergo laparoscopic surgery. To test efficacy, one might look at a simple short term outcome such as the success rate of ductal clearance. When considering effectiveness however, one is challenging not merely the intervention but the policy of using this intervention. Such a study would now have to involve all patients with bile duct stones, some of whom might not be fit for laparoscopic surgery. In addition, effectiveness involves consideration of a wider spectrum of outcomes, such as survival and quality of life. Surgical papers regularly confuse these issues. Be sure that you can recognise this confusion when it occurs.

How was the study conducted? Case series, before and after studies and randomised controlled trials, probably represent an order of ascending scientific merit but even in a controlled trial, you need to think about how patients were chosen and allocated.

Who was studied? Demographic data may be important. Was the study based on a small local population or individuals referred to a tertiary centre? Does the study represent the full spectrum of a disease? Are there clear inclusion and exclusion criteria?

What intervention and outcome measures were used? Compliance is important in most studies. Withdrawals, dropouts, crossovers and poor compliers all need to be considered, to see how much influence these factors might have had on the final results. For instance, consider oesophageal cancer and the role of neo-adjuvant chemoradiation followed by oesophagectomy and how results might be expressed in terms of outcome. Let us assume we begin with one hundred patients with this diagnosis and that 40% of them are eligible for this treatment. In these patients, assume a drop-out rate of 10% due to chemoradiation toxicity and a 6% mortality at that stage. Add a further 6% mortality after surgery. Presume that 50% of the surgical survivors had complete pathological responses in the resected specimen and that 75% of these are the only patients alive after three years. Now consider outcome measures. Expressed as overall survival for oesophageal cancer at three years, this is 12% (12/100) but it could be 30% (12/40) for the patients receiving multi-modal therapy on an 'intention to treat' basis, 37.5% (12/32) for those who actually received the treatment and were not killed by it or even 75% (12/16) of those with a complete pathological response. Be sure that you are not hoodwinked by the style of reporting outcome!

How many, refers to statistical significance and sample size. The most important question here is, did the authors consider the methods of analysis and necessary sample size before they started the study? Watch out for the popular trick of carrying out multiple analyses on a data set. This increases the likelihood that a significant result will be obtained by chance alone. Small sample size leads to trials with weak power to detect important differences in outcome. The so-called Type II statistical error is common in surgical papers, where the study is too small to detect statistically significant differences.

At the end of a paper, you must ask the question, so what? Is all of this of any real significance? A statistical increase in survival with chemotherapy for patients with advanced pancreas cancer may only need to be a few weeks, but is it really important or worthwhile?

Review articles require the same type of critical appraisal. There is a special issue here. Look out for the introduction of bias imposed by selectivity on the part of the author.

Writer's Block

'Clear writers, like clear fountains, do not seem as deep as they are'
Walter Savage Landor

By now you will have begun to formulate ideas and hopefully have an outline in mind. You will probably begin with 'writer's block' but surprisingly this is not a bad thing, as it inhibits the generation of ill considered spontaneous rubbish. Writer's block may be a form of internal criticism, where the words selected to express an idea are censored before they reach the page. It is a major problem for 'perfectionists' because it restricts the ability to formulate ideas in written words, even when such individuals have a clear grasp of these ideas. Thankfully it can actually be used to your advantage if you can switch it off in the manuscript drafting phase and switch it back on when editing.

Your first writing task is to create an outline which will lead to a first draft of the final paper. There is no need to be inhibited by writer's block at this stage because these words and phrases are unlikely to appear in the final document. The production of the outline can be achieved in a number of ways, usually as a flow chart with arrows leading from one point to the next or in a hub and spoke fashion around a central theme. Ultimately, it is no more than the list of those points which you collected during your literature appraisal that you feel still need to be included in the final document. There is no need at this stage to be unduly concerned by language. It is from this draft outline that you can start to deal with sections of the paper. It is best to start with the easiest sections first rather than trying to go through the paper in a fixed order of introduction, methods, results and discussion. Methods and results are generally easier to write than the other sections. Tackling these may help to overcome writer's block. All of this helps the author to develop a flow of ideas, enabling the writer to convey a logical train of thought to the reader. It is now that you have to give some thought to the actual words and develop a writing style. The latter is discussed in detail in Chapter 7 but a few fundamental points are worthy of emphasis here:

- Keep sentences short.

- Use short words if possible - 'simple' not 'elementary'.

- Use the correct word properly - 'data', a plural word meaning accepted facts based on calculations.

- Avoid neologisms - 'speech' not 'verbalisation'.

- Keep away from double negatives - 'it is not unlike ....'.

- Avoid clichés - 'like the plague!'

Only at this point are you ready to deal with the specific issues in writing the actual manuscript.

Commentary
by N. S. Williams
Professor of Surgery, The Royal London Hospital, London, UK

Derek Alderson provides valuable advice to the fledgling author, all of which should be heeded. This author wishes only to add snippets garnered from his own experience, which might provide additional help. Professor Alderson mentions self-imposed deadlines, but beware of the editorially imposed deadline. If you are asked to contribute an article to a prestigious publication you will naturally be flattered, but do not let this initial euphoria allow you to accept the assignment if there is no way you can comply with the date of delivery. Pressure from the editor will inevitably come and make your life a misery. Some of the best friendships have been mightily stretched by failure to meet a deadline.

Structuring an article depends on the type that is being written. An original research paper tends to write itself. The hypothesis, methods and data are all there; it is only the interpretation of that data that presents the difficulties. Reviews need to explore the literature thoroughly. However, they need to be critical yet balanced. Chapters are daunting and need to be broken down into sections, which are more manageable. Whatever article is being written, remember that science is international and the bibliography should mirror this. There are some individuals who believe that if a fellow countryman did not write the article, it is not worth quoting. Even if one is foolish enough to believe this, keep in mind that a referee is very likely to be a 'foreigner'!

Chapter
5

Chapter 6

Writing

a

manuscript

S. A. Wells, Jr.

Professor of Surgery

Duke University School of Medicine

DUMC, Durham

NC, U.S.A.

Writing well is difficult, particularly when it comes to scientific topics, since the subject is complex and often of interest only to a limited audience. However, there are many examples of good scientific writing, the skill being to convey one's message simply so that it is easily understood and absorbed by the reader. A published body of work, whether performed in the laboratory or the clinic, should be looked on as an academic currency. Aspiring basic or clinical scientists feel an enormous pressure to establish themselves as accomplished clinical or laboratory investigators, realizing that academic promotion, election to membership of distinguished societies, and consideration for senior leadership positions at prestigious institutions are largely determined by an evaluation of a candidate's publications. Often young scientists place undue emphasis on the number of scientific publications, rather than the quality. However, discerning promotion, selection or search committees, charged with judging a candidate's worth, rarely confuse quantity and quality. Therefore, much thought should be given to what to write and where to publish the work, as a permanent record is being established that will represent one's academic accomplishments.

Types of manuscript

Surgical articles are usually written in one of three forms: case reports of a clinical observation, scientific reviews and original scientific articles based on either laboratory or clinical research. Whatever the form, one should strive for clarity, remembering that scientific writing is by necessity highly structured and thinly prosaic. If the study is well designed, the methodology appropriate for the experiment, and the results clear, the author's work should be relatively easy.

The case report

Some surgeons find a clinical case of great interest and decide to record it, usually in the form of a 'case report and review of the literature'. Clinical case reports are usually the work of young authors and represent an early attempt at medical publication. These articles rarely signal an important clinical advance and many medical editors do not consider them for publication. Above all, case reports should be brief and carefully illustrated to emphasize the primary and hopefully novel observation.

The review article

In these publications there is a review of a single topic. The manuscripts are usually lengthy, and analyse or summarize a body of previously published work, although some authors include data from their clinic or laboratory as part of the report. The reader finds these articles valuable when seeking a broad overview of a given topic. Well written reviews take time and necessitate a careful study of the relevant literature. The task is particularly challenging when the author attempts to clarify a controversial issue.

The original scientific publication

These articles provide the backbone for the advancement of medical knowledge and represent the first line of scientific publications. The importance of an original scientific article is directly related to the quality of the experimental data on which it is based. The more important the hypothesis being tested, the better the experimental design, and the more definitive the results of the experiment, the easier it is to write the paper.

Original scientific articles usually have a standard structure consisting of: an abstract, an introduction, materials and methods, results, and the discussion. In planning the manuscript one begins with a careful analysis of the study results, as an objective review of the data will define what conclusions can be drawn. How the author handles the discussion of the materials and methods is a function of the writer's intellect and style, but it is important not to make the common mistake of drawing conclusions beyond what is defined by the results of the experimental data.

The abstract

The abstract is a brief description of the study. More commonly, structured abstracts are being used to state: the principal objectives and scope of the investigation, the methodology used, the experimental results and the conclusions of the study. The well prepared abstract enables the readers to grasp the essence of the study, to decide whether it is relevant to their interests and to determine whether the article is worth reading. The importance of the abstract is greater in the current era of online search machines, when abstracts are so readily available and retrievable. Abstracts should give an overview of the study and not exceed 250 words. Even though the abstract is the part of the article first seen by the reader, it should be written after the rest of the manuscript is completed.

The introduction

The author provides a background for the reader by defining the problem to be addressed and discussing the pertinent literature. The author might find it necessary to describe generally one or more experimental methods used in the study. The introduction is occasionally concluded with a brief statement about the results of the study but this is controversial and some authors choose to leave the important findings to the discussion.

The materials and methods

It is important that the author describe the subjects of the study, whether humans or laboratory animals, and the clinical or laboratory methods employed. If human subjects were involved it should be stated that an institutional review board approved the study. It is frequently impractical to explain a laboratory method in detail, in which case a reference to a previously published description suffices. The statistical methods should be described and referenced.

This section of the manuscript tends to be rather dry but the information is critical to the paper and precision is essential. During editorial review of the manuscript this section is evaluated carefully to determine whether the reviewer understands the methodology sufficiently to repeat the experiment. Often, one or more methods described in this section have not been reported previously and will serve as the basis for future laboratory experiments by other investigators. It is particularly important that this section be clear and uncluttered because it provides the basis for all that follows.

Clinical studies may lend themselves only to a report of a series of patients evaluated over a long period of time. If it can be achieved, the most important design of a clinical study is the prospective randomized controlled trial. With this method one obtains study groups that are balanced with regard to known baseline factors and presumably to unknown factors as well. No other study design accomplishes this. It is dismaying to see how many clinical studies compare historical controls, or a matched set of patients as controls, or even no controls, to the study group, rather than follow the more meaningful design provided by a prospective randomized trial.

The results

This section represents the heart of the manuscript and may be very short if the preceding materials and methods section, and the succeeding discussion section, are well written. The results can often be expressed in tabular form and it is not necessary to present all of the experimental data, just that which is relevant. If there is any part of the manuscript that demands crispness and clarity it is the results section as it represents new knowledge derived from the investigation.

One must guard against redundancy in the results section. Do not repeat in the text data that are also presented in tables or figures and do not amplify the materials and methods section in the results section.

The discussion

The purpose here is to provide an analytical interpretation of the results and to state what principles and relationships are learned. One must be careful to interpret the results yet not repeat them. In many instances it will be important to state how the experimental data contrast and compare with the results of previously reported studies. In the final section of the discussion one should state the conclusions of the study and summarize the evidence for each of them. The discussion flows directly from the sections on materials and methods and results, and it is important that there be logic to the relationship. Do not hesitate to point out any weakness in the study. Prophylactic self-criticism pre-empts readership criticism.

Authorship

Little has been said about the listing of authors but this is an important matter as it is often the source of conflict. The authors should be listed in the order in which they most contributed to the study. In some centres it has been customary for the head of a laboratory to be listed as the last author on all papers published from the group. It is my strong view that the persons primarily involved in the research should get the credit, especially younger scientists who frequently have the original idea for the study and perform most of the work. The duty of the senior scientist is to provide an intellectual milieu for younger investigators and to create an opportunity for them to grow and gain intellectual independence. Nevertheless, there are often arguments about the sequence in which contributors are listed on manuscripts and resolution of this conflict rests with the senior scientist in the laboratory where the work was performed. Trouble can usually be avoided if decisions about listing priority of authors have been taken early in the study and certainly before writing the paper. Remember that some journals limit the number of authors.

With time and practice one can master the art of writing scientific papers. Above all, it should be remembered that substance is paramount and without significant data flowing from a well designed study the style of the article will be irrelevant.

Commentary
by D. M. Dent
Professor of Surgery, Head of Department, Department of Surgery, Faculty of Health Sciences, University of Cape Town, Cape Town, South Africa.

Drawing from his experience in scientific publication, Dr Wells provides sound advice to the aspirant author. I agree that it is the quality and not the quantity of publications that enhance a CV, or any scientific endeavor for that matter. Many Institutions, including my own, dauntingly ask applicants for what they consider to be their best four publications, the reasons why they chose them, and how frequently they have been cited. Dr Wells also provides an example of clarity and economy in scientific writing.

I agree that small species such as the case report is becoming rare and is due for extinction. While our surgical grandfathers published the monstrous, or the extraordinarily coincidental, and embryonic surgeons used this format for their earliest literary attempts (frequently as a foot in the door for a review), few journals now accept them. It is unlikely that the tide of surgery is advanced by an account of an unfortunate patient: 'Testicular torsion presenting with vertical nystagmus in a patient with Marfan's syndrome.'

Reviews provide comprehensive up-to-date information on single topics and eclipse chapters in books, which are frequently dated and repetitive with successive editions. The New England Journal of Medicine, the Lancet and the British Journal of Surgery provide valuable examples. The essence of a good review is that it be written by an authority in the subject, with a grasp of what is important and what not; of what is fact, and what is speculation. The review section of a thesis (blood and sweat that it was), does not easily find itself suitable for this sort of publication.

I support Dr Wells' contention that the scientific article is the backbone for the advancement of medical knowledge. He stresses the importance of the abstract, which should encapsulate the entire article and which exactingly tests the art of crystallization. It is the shibboleth for acceptance or rejection. Dr Wells then explores each of the components of the Bradford Hill construct: The introduction (whatever it was that was preying on the author's mind prompting them to start the work) should be a perfect counterfoil to the results and conclusion. The problem should be posed, and that, and that only, amplified in the discussion in the light of what was found. The methods section is vital, and it is here that the reviewer sharpens their scrutiny. The initial premise, or analytic technique may be fatally flawed, and this flaw will run like a San Andreas fault through the entire article. Invalid comparison (to disparate groups, to others, or to the past) is probably the most common error in publication. The prospective trial with its rigor of eligibility, proformas, the recording of all events and their dispassionate analysis has changed what is now regarded as 'evidence', and the prospective researcher and author is well advised to plan their methods in detail before embarking on the work.

The medical literary buffet groans with journals and articles, and the dyspeptic public - and reviewers - demand quality. Dr Wells describes how to achieve this.

Chapter
6

Chapter 7

Advice

on

writing style

J. R. Farndon

Professor and Head of Division

University of Bristol

&

Consultant Surgeon

Bristol Royal Infirmary, Bristol, UK.

> *'Those who write as they speak,*
> *even though they speak well, write badly.'*
> **Comte de Buffon, Discours sur le style, 1753**

Why does it matter how we write. Surely it should not matter so long as the message is transmitted, received, assimilated and acted upon.

Would you prefer a Rolls Royce or a Skoda? Both may be silent in overdrive and well able to maintain 70mph day after day but the images of the cars on the highway transmit different messages.

Depiction of a scene by Raphael (16 Century) will differ from Rubens (17 C), from Reynolds (18 C), from Rousseau (19 C), from Roberts (20 C). We might enjoy the imagery of Debussy, the precision and complexity of Chopin or the lyrical spontaneity of Poulenc. These are all forms in their own right. Surgical writing has its own form - or should have. Journals have neither the space nor resource to allow impressionistic writing; readers do not have time to search for the main theme and writers, readers and publishers should care about quality at all times. Yes, you could rush the words onto the page, you could spend time developing themes, you could hide the message in ornate text, you could repeat phrases but …… don't! Like surgery itself, surgeons appreciate things which are clean, objective and precise. This should apply to your writing.

Some style matters may be described in 'instructions to authors' or in instructions from the book publisher. Do read them carefully and try to follow them closely. Their adoption adds a uniformity and quality to the product as a whole.

The Title

This should give a clear message about the article's content - it should be as short as possible and without colons, semicolons, hyphens or question marks. It should indicate the nature of the study. It should not use gimmicks - we would prefer to read 'A comparative study of scissors versus diathermy in the treatment of patients with haemorrhoids' rather than 'Scissors and diathermy both bring haemorrhoids to a painful tail end'! It should avoid direct reference to animals if these were used since, in some countries, animal rights activists search out and attack scientists who carry out such work. Attribution is not required in titles - the institute and authors are clearly defined elsewhere in the text. That is, avoid 'One thousand patients with ingrowing toenails - the Gasworks General Hospital experience'.

So 'Laparoscopic or open cholecystectomy: a comparative study of 12,000 patients carried out in St Murdo's General Hospital, Trumpton-by-Sea, in a prospective and blind manner' becomes 'A prospective, blind comparative study of open versus laparoscopic cholecystectomy' and 'The effect of a Sandostatin analogue on the incidence of multi-organ failure in a Taurine-induced model of acute pancreatitis in the New Zealand marmoset' becomes 'Sandostatin analogue reduces the incidence of multi-organ failure in an experimental model of acute pancreatitis'. Note this latter title is shorter, direct, gives results and avoids the reference to animals. The verb is declaratory.

It is important that the key elements of the work feature in title words to ensure appropriate search mechanisms and engines identify the appropriate articles. Prospective randomised studies need to be so labelled to ensure identification by appropriate databases such as Cochrane.

The Abstract

The abstract or summary of the article or chapter must follow author instructions exactly. Most abstracts will be structured with a word limit. Your sentences may have to be even more crisp and to the point. Abbreviations may be used but need to be characterised in both abstract and full text at first use.

The Introduction

This should be brief, quickly set the scene for the work to be described and pose the questions to be answered or the hypothesis to be tested. If your paper examines xenotransplantation of sheep islets to cure diabetes in man then we do not need to begin with the first description of diabetes in the Ebers Papyrus. Begin with the latest work on islet xenotransplantation. Make your question or hypothesis the culmination of this section. For example: 'This work examines the effect of cyclosporine alone on the immune response of patients with diabetes to isolated sheep islets transplanted into the spleen.'

- Keep your style tight and economical.

  'It has been said that xenotransplantation will soon suffer the adverse events of the processes of immune rejection' becomes 'Xenotransplants suffer early immunological rejection'.

- Avoid elitism and triumphalism.

  'The studies were carried out in St Murdo's General Hospital, which is a tertiary referral centre, and the procedures were all carried out by AHPS during his 25 years as the senior surgeon.' What is the definition of a tertiary referral centre? Who gives the certificate for such a centre? Is the credibility of the work dependent upon skills peculiar to Professor AHPS? Is the duration of the study of any interest or relevance? Does it really matter that the work was done at St Murdo's? We can read the affiliation separately.

◆ Exceptions to affiliation details, who operated and when occur when these variables themselves are under study or relate to the observations you make. For example, it may be an important distinction that all the procedures described were carried out by a single surgeon rather than any member of the team who happened to be on call. The quality of these results may depend upon the skills so developed by a surgeon operating upon ingrowing toe nails only for 25 years!

◆ Personal pronouns can and should be avoided if possible. 'We were the first to show that sheep to human pancreatic islet xenotransplants are rejected within seven days' is better as 'Sheep to human islet transplants are rejected within seven days' (reference). The reference allows the reader to see who first described this exciting, unexpected observation in 1913! Leave it to the readers to determine whether you were first since there will be someone out there who did it five years before you did. Leave it to the readers to determine whether your study was the first randomised trial of islet xenotransplants because someone will have just published the first trial in 'Transplantation'.

Materials and methods

If your work is clinical then write about 'people' or 'patients'. 'Cases' are for wine. Being described as a case is demeaning. What are cancer patients? What are colorectal cancer patients? or infected patients? This is sloppy writing. Better 'patients with colorectal cancer'. If the descriptive is long and complex then patients can be gathered together into groups. Group A comprised 25 patients with cirrhosis, infected venous ulcers and gallstones. Group B comprised 26 patients with cirrhosis, infected venous ulcers but no gallstones.

Avoid tables giving individual patient details - the data can often be summarised in text or a table, e.g.:

TABLE 1
Group A Details

	12 men	13 women
Age Range (years)	17-36	19-45
Bilirubin Range (nmol/l)	50-110	73-140
Mean area of venous ulcer (sq cm)	45.5	36.3

Patient initials, dates of birth, record numbers and addresses must never be used as these could lead to patient identification.

Ethical and humanitarian issues must always be included whether your paper deals with humans or animals.

In methods, use references as often as you can to previously reported methods or techniques. If there is no difference in the method you used you need say no more than 'Sheep islet antibodies were measured by the technique described by Buggins et al (ref).' Avoid saying '... described by Buggins et al (ref) which, in brief, involved washing a set of test tubes in distilled water and setting these in racks of twelve. Antibody was then diluted 1 : 10,000 with phosphate buffered saline. Antibody was detected by an anti-antibody raised in rabbits against sheep islets ... etc, etc'. There is no need for this detail. Allow the reference to do the work.

Be sure to give the number of subjects, the variance of the variables measured, the precision of the methods of measurement, the intra- and inter-observer variance, the power calculations used to determine the number of experiments. Describe the statistics to be used in the analysis. Don't just say the results were analysed on a computer!

Abbreviations are often first used in an introduction but can become more prominent in the methods section. Always characterise an abbreviation in full at first use as: infected venous ulcers (IVU). Avoid unnecessary and frequent abbreviations since the text can become cluttered and uncomfortable to read. 'Twenty-five patients with Type I diabetes mellitus (TIDM), cirrhosis, infected venous ulcers (IVU) and gallstones (GS) received $2x10^6$ isolated sheep islets of Langerhaus (ISIL) by direct intrasplenic needle injection (DINI)'. These abbreviations are confusing, difficult to remember and not necessary. Textual abbreviations can be used and once characterised in full you could write only about 'islets' or 'ulcers' because your readers will have appreciated the subject of your paper and will know that you would not mislead by suddenly writing or thinking about guinea pig islets or duodenal ulcers!

Results

This is one section where you need to avoid duplicate or triplicate effort. Text may be very brief because results can be given in tables or figures. Determine which format will best transmit this very important part of your paper or book chapter. Do not feel you need to emphasise the importance of your results by presenting them in figures, tables and describing them fully in the text. The editor is likely to ask you to present your results in one format only. You need to decide which format will best suit the complexity and range of your results. Be sure that the legends for your figures or tables are as crisp and precise as your overall title.

Avoid interpretation and discussion of the results in this section.

Do not use techniques to make results appear more credible - 30 percent sounds very impressive but two out of six probably means nothing. Do not bother to use percentage terms if the experimental number is less than 50 - just give the absolute numbers.

Do not feel that you must apply statistics. An observational study of 50 patients with infected venous ulcers does not need statistical analysis. Fuller Albright was one of the first to say - 'If you need statistics I don't believe it'.

Discussion

The magic 'economy' word continues to apply. Discuss your results in relation to your introductory question or hypothesis and in the context of previously cited work in your introduction. Do not be tempted to write a comprehensive review. Rather be sure that your reader knows whether your hypothesis is proved or disproved.

This is another section in which to avoid elite triumphalism: 'We at St Murdo's, in 2,500 experiments of sheep to guinea pig allografts, were the first to show that such xenotransplants do not work' becomes 'This work shows that sheep to guinea pig xenotransplants reject within two days'.

Other articles - Leaders, Reviews, Editorials

Leaders and editorials often allow some licence in style. Of necessity there is often a limit on length and number of references, e.g. 1000 words and five references for a *BJS* leader. Some political spin may be acceptable but the style is expected to be authoritative and opinionated.

Reviews and systematic reviews will have specific instructions. The methodology of gathering material for reviews must be carefully described. If you draw upon the text of previously published reviews be careful not to 'lift' too much text into your own writing without appropriate reference or acknowledgement. The cut-off point for plagiarism is getting smaller.

A few brief guidelines

Structure

- Try and keep your sentences within 15-20 words.

- Use language that will be understood by the readership.

- Choose your verb carefully - be sure to use a verb. For example, 'Ingrowing toe nails are common and painful when they occur on the littlest toe. The fourth toe resembling the most lateral toe'. The last sentence must either be 'The fourth toe resembles the most lateral toe' or 'The fourth toe, resembling the most lateral toe, can also be affected by ingrowth'.

- Avoid split infinitives. For example, 'to operate' is an infinitive. You might just get away with 'to fearlessly operate' but perhaps not 'to fearlessly, remorselessly and tirelessly operate'. The natural flow of words might allow the split, for example, 'to carefully consider'.

- Avoid discursive preface remarks such has 'It has long been held that ....'

- Try and think of economical ways of saying the same thing. 'At this moment in time' becomes 'Currently' or 'Now'. Some phrases have become clichés so 'few and far between' means 'rare'. Tautology is saying the same thing twice over in different words, e.g. 'A searching enquiry into the causes of pancreatitis'. Could a surgical enquiry into the causes of pancreatitis be anything but searching?

- In correspondence try and be direct while retaining civility. There is no need for everyone to say they enjoyed reading the article by Buggins only then to be fiercely critical of everything which Buggins did. Why not say at the outset: 'We attempted to repeat the method of Buggins but found .....'

Punctuation

Full stops should be your main punctuation mark. The other marks can be used in scientific writing but are less essential than in prose or poetry. Commas will be used to separate lists - e.g. 'The causes of pancreatitis include: gallstones, alcohol, hypercalcaemia and genetic factors.' Note the use of the colon to introduce a list. This mark will be used occasionally in your writing and mainly in this function. Commas also separate parts of a sentence and, by their position, can lend emphasis or poise to the sentence. Note their use in the sentence you have just read.

The semicolon ';' is likely to appear less often in your writing and if you are ever tempted to use it think whether a full stop would do as well. The semicolon should be separating two sentences which could stand alone but which must be closely related. An example: 'Hyperparathyroidism is rare in the general population; it occurs more frequently in women.' The semicolon is also useful as a separator of complex items in a list, e.g. 'Cushing's syndrome may be caused by a pituitary adenoma secreting ACTH; an adenoma of the adrenal gland producing excess cortisol; a tumour producing ectopic ACTH; and liver disease producing pseudo-Cushing's syndrome'. An alternative in vogue is the use of bullet points, for example - 'Cushing's syndrome may be caused by:

- a pituitary adenoma secreting ACTH.

- an adenoma of the adrenal gland producing excess cortisol, etc'.

This style is particularly useful if the listed items are more complex than a single phrase or sentence.

Your most likely use of parenthesis (round brackets such as those around these nine words) will be to remove an abbreviation or acronym out of the mainstream of the sentence and must always be used this way at first characterisation of the abbreviation. For example, 'extra corporeal shock wave lithotripsy (ECSWL) can be used to fragment renal and biliary stones'. Do not so characterise an abbreviation if you are not going to use it frequently in subsequent text. Use parenthesis to cordon off an aside or supplementary text, e.g. 'Severe, acute pancreatitis (presence of more than five risk factors) is associated with a mortality of 30%'.

Brackets are, strictly speaking, square and are used within round brackets or to show interpolation. For example, 'Pancreatitis can be caused by gall stones or consumption of excess alcohol (beer, whisky [single malt or blend], wine or porter)'.

The apostrophe can be confusing to native English writers and might be a nightmare to contributors not using English frequently. In its possessive function add '-'s' except if the possessor ends in an '-s'. So, it is Cushing's syndrome but Graves' disease. Confusions easily occur. If the possessor ends in 's' then '-'s' or just a final apostrophe are equally correct. More confusion can occur in other functions of the apostrophe. It should be used to show a missing letter e.g. 'don't' is really 'do not'. In scientific writing 'don't' would be sloppy style anyway. 'It's' bad form to use this instead of 'it is' but editors will use red pens for corrections. A journal takes <u>its</u> responsibilities very seriously in ensuring that sufficient red pen is used. In this last sentence 'its' responsibilities is a pronoun usage and is a single possessive pronoun in its own right without apostrophes.

Ellipsis ....; quotation marks ' ' or ' '; exclamation marks !; and question marks ? should not be required in surgical writing. The reference system allows attribution of ideas, methods and historical concepts. If you use text verbatim from a previously published article or book then this must be marked as such by quotation marks as well as reference source.

Words

Spellings - do check whether you are sending your work to an American or British journal or publisher. Common differences in spellings / nomenclature are:

American English	British English
Operating room	Theatre
Anesthesiologist	Anaesthetist
Sulfur	Sulphur
Maneuver	Manoeuvre
Practice	Practise (verb)
Esophagus	Oesophagus
Tumor	Tumour

American spellings favour verbs to be spelled with a 'z' - e.g. standardize.

Data are plural. **A number** is plural. **The number** is singular.

Gender

Try and write in a gender neutral way except when the disease or study is gender specific and then write about 'men and women' not 'males and females'.

Avoid using 'he', 'his' or 'him' if at all possible. The same applies for the female counterparts. 'S/he' or 'he/she' looks clumsy and cannot be spoken easily. It is sometimes possible to use the plural 'they' or a collective noun such as 'surgeons' or 'patients' to avoid the gender issue.

Some pet hates

'Whilst' is archaic - use 'while' if you must.

Must you use 'among' or 'amongst'? Try 'of'.

'In toto' can be replaced by 'completely' or 'entirely'.

'Editress' is now defunct and replaced by the accepted unisex term 'Editor'.

Conclusion

Style does matter. It is the final polish on your work. Whether as first, intermediate or last author take this aspect of your work seriously and, acknowledging that skills in writing are not universally distributed in surgeons, do not be ashamed or diffident about using your red pen. Until all learning occurs from a screen or subliminally enjoy the feel of paper and enjoy the craft of writing stylishly.

Useful Texts

'The Plain English Guide' - Martin Cutts. Oxford University Press, Oxford and New York.

'Everyman's Good English Guide' - Harry Fieldhouse. JM Dent & Sons Ltd, London, Melbourne and Toronto.

Commentary
by W. B. Campbell
Consultant Surgeon and Honorary Professor, Royal Devon and Exeter Hospital, Exeter, UK.

This discourse on writing style is as thorough and masterful as one might expect from as experienced an author and journal editor as John Farndon. Few others could incorporate Rubens, a Skoda, the Ebers Papyrus and the Gasworks General Hospital in the same piece.

Attention to the basics - observing journal requirements; a crisp clear style; and proper use of punctuation - simply deserve repetition and emphasis. However, the latter sentence illustrates two points I would argue - use of semicolons (to separate parallel phrases more emphatically than with commas) and his neglect of the humble dash. Another point some authors need to learn is the use of paragraphs: the task of a reviewer is made particularly gloomy by whole pages of text without paragraph breaks.

I would add advice about the Abstract and the Discussion. Remember that many people only read the Abstract of a paper: be sure to include in it all the results and main messages you particularly want to convey. Writing a good Discussion is an art, but I advocate one basic rule. Make a list of the points you want to discuss; write a succinct paragraph on each; then place them in the most logical order. Craft a 'strong finish'.

The Results certainly should not duplicate information in the Tables, but may benefit from reference to the most important observations contained in them.

Master craftsmen all have personal foibles, and John Farndon is no exception, with his dislike of colons in titles and his incomprehension of 'colorectal cancer patients'. That said, I fully agree with all his 'pet hates'!

Chapter 8

The 'foreign' author

M. Rothmund

Professor and Chairman
Department of Surgery, Philipps-University
Marburg, Germany

A. Fingerhut

Chief of Service, Digestive Surgery, Centre Hospitalier
Intercommunal, Poissy, France & Associate Professor of Surgery
Louisiana State University Medical School
New Orleans, LA, U.S.A.

Throughout the history of medicine several languages have been the 'lingua franca'. English is likely to remain the language of medicine and science despite the fact that more people worldwide speak Chinese, Hindi or other languages. The main reasons are the ease of learning and understanding basic English, the predominance of English usage in the medical community, the role of English as the main language on the Internet and in electronic and traditional publishing. Here, the 'foreign' author is therefore defined as one whose mother language is not English.

Why English?

Why does a 'foreign' author want to publish in English? The answer to this question is simple: no one in the scientific world publishes data for the unselfish purpose of advancing science and medicine alone. There are always more reasons for publishing, the most important being promotion in one's own academic career. A French, German or Japanese surgeon who has produced new and important data could be called 'naive' or even 'silly' by friends and colleagues if the article were sent to a national journal. Studies by the Institute of Scientific Information have shown that the majority of all scientific literature is written and published in English and that the English language literature is by far the most cited. According to impact factor ratings, an English publication will be cited on average 3.7 times, whereas German, French and Japanese publications will be cited only 0.6, 0.5 and 0.5 times respectively. An article written in English attracts a greater than sixfold higher response than, for example, an article written in German [1]. This means that the diffusion of knowledge and the recognition of the authors among peers are greatly enhanced if the work is published in English.

The foreign author who knows English

Speaking and writing proper English is therefore a prerequisite for making a straightforward academic career for almost all non-English-speaking scientists. Many promising academic surgeons from non-English-speaking countries spend time in hospitals or research centres in the USA, UK or Canada and have an opportunity to learn (medical) English. For most, reliance on remembered school English is often insufficient to allow fluent speech or writing in English.

The 'foreign' author should always ask a native English-speaking colleague to review the final draft of a manuscript, especially first papers. An acknowledgement at the end of the article should be sufficient to thank the colleague for efforts in simple translation.

The foreign author who does not know English

The 'foreign' author who has not expanded language skills beyond basic English always has to rely on a colleague to translate the article or on a professional translator. The first choice is undoubtedly the best. Experiences with commercial translators may be disappointing, expensive, and the meaning and message of the manuscript may be altered or lost in the translation, simply because most translators lack adequate comprehension of medical subtleties. A further problem is the secretarial task. The surgeon writer may not be capable of typing or may have to ask for secretarial assistance, for which the same language problems might arise. Perfectly bilingual secretaries are more scarce than perfectly bilingual surgeons.

Some international journals provide editorial assistance to optimize the English style of a manuscript; such an example is the *World Journal of Surgery*. This does not mean that these journals are able to rewrite manuscripts into proper English, and it is obviously very important to prepare a manuscript in the best English style possible.

While most journals do not accept or refuse papers from foreign authors on the basis of 'good' or 'poor' English, proper English does lead to easier comprehension, more effective refereeing and editing, and therefore expedites publication.

To publish nationally, internationally or both?

Most non-English-speaking authors want not only to promote their academic careers and be known internationally but also to be known and to advance in their careers in their own country, and publication in their national language is mandatory. It is still a fact that in countries with fairly large populations, such as Japan, Germany, France and Italy, most native clinicians read and gather information from journals written in their own language. The non-English-speaking author sometimes has to make a difficult decision concerning the aims and objectives of the manuscript [2]: should the paper promote the academic career and international recognition, or should it contribute to national reputation? Non-English-speaking authors may be divided into two groups: those who publish exclusively in their native language, achieve an average or below-average academic career and work in a non-academic or teaching hospital. The second group is composed of those who place publications both internationally and nationally; these surgeons usually become chiefs of university departments of affiliated hospitals. There are few, if any, who will publish exclusively in English. This is true for basic scientists only.

There are important economic and academic considerations from the perspective of national non-English journals. If authors send all good manuscripts to English journals, the national language publications may wither as they publish only second-class original data or review papers only. National journals try to overcome this situation by providing excellent English abstracts and listing in international publication retrieval systems. In the near future, electronic publication of an English translation of the full text may be practical and, in this way, duplicate publications will also disappear.

In order to avoid decline in its performance, the publishers of *Langenbecks Archiv für Chirurgie*, a German-language journal founded in 1860, decided in 1998 to publish exclusively in English. The hope was to increase the impact factor (which indeed happened) and to attract good manuscripts from German authors who would otherwise have sent material to 'English' journals. Time will show whether the journal succeeds in this effort.

Duplicate publication in a foreign language: is it redundant?

Previously some authors have published the same material concurrently in their national language and in English because of the difference in impact factors of the respective journals and insufficiencies in the indexing system. In the electronic age this is no longer possible as the new databases will index practically all articles (usually with an English translation of the title). If potential (foreign) authors continue to do this without informing the editors of both journals, they fulfil the criteria for duplicate publication, a serious and dishonest situation which is rightly viewed as a publishing misdemeanour. The present authors think that this problem should be eliminated by discussion and agreement among established editors of the most important medical journals worldwide. The Vancouver group [3] in 1997 published prerequisites that would allow duplicate publication, particularly in two different languages. The conditions that should be met are [3]:

- 'The authors must have received approval from the editors of both journals. The editors concerned with secondary publication must have a photocopy, reprint or manuscript of the primary version.

- The priority of the primary publication is respected by a publication interval by at least one week (unless specifically negotiated otherwise by both editors).

- The paper for secondary publication is intended for a different group of readers; an abbreviated version would be sufficient.

- The secondary version reflects faithfully the data and interpretation of the primary version.

◆ A footnote on the title page of the secondary version informs readers, peers and documenting agencies that the paper has been published in whole or in part in the primary reference. A suitable footnote might read: 'This article is based on a study first reported in: (title of journal, with full reference).'

◆ Permission for such secondary publication should be free of charge.'

If journals worldwide would agree to these conditions, non-English-speaking authors would be freed from a dilemma: should I publish important data in a national language journal of which my peers outside the country will not take note with almost no impact points, or should I publish in an English journal with gain of more impact points for my academic career even though my national peers and national institutions will not be aware of the paper? English-language journals should accept the above-mentioned conditions and should not always demand to be the principal journal for publication, relegating the national journals to second position.

Finally, important papers in national (non-English) journals do not easily find the correct path to the citation index or into overviews and meta-analyses (Egger Lancet 1997). This deficit should hopefully be overcome in the latest electronic publishing era.

References

1   Garfield E, Willjams-Dorof A. Language use in national research: a citation analysis. *Current Contents* 1990; 33: 5-17.

2   Rothmund M, Bartsch D, Lorenz W. Where should you publish your paper? In: Troidl H *et al*, eds. *Surgical Research*. Heidelberg: Springer, 1997: 119-26.

3   International Committee of Medical Journal, eds. Uniform requirements for manuscripts submitted to biomedical journals. *N Engl J Med* 1997; 336: 309-15.

Commentary
by R. Saadia

Charles William Burns Professor of Trauma Surgery,
The University of Manitoba, Winnipeg, Canada.

The preeminence of English in medical publishing is a fact of academic life and I fully agree with the views expressed by Professors Rothmund and Fingerhut. The topic of the 'foreign' author does open a Pandora's box since 'foreign' authors do not hold the monopoly of poor English. Consider the following sentence gleaned, in my recent reading, from a highly-rated surgical journal: 'Although there is no shotgun (authors' emphasis) approach to blood component transfusion therapy, the coagulopathy shown by these patients has a time course that is more rapid than stat (sic) laboratories can presently keep up with'. The authors names are impeccably anglo-saxon, yet even I had to steady my 'foreign' nerves in order to continue my reading. The paper was couched in a consistently inelegant style - but otherwise was sound enough. Give me 'Turkish' or 'Italian English' any time!

Is the 'foreign' paper at a disadvantage in the peer-review process? I suspect some (very few) referees still cling to certain atavistic prejudices in equating 'foreign' with 'inferior'. This is not a significant problem currently. Editors enlist much 'foreign' expertise to help vet submitted material. Certainly prospective 'foreign' authors should never be discouraged from presenting their work in English; and having faced a rejection, they are quite entitled to invoke xenophobia ... only if the pain is unbearable! Nonetheless, it is not surprising that a sloppy style or too many gross mistakes inevitably cast doubts about the rigour of the research itself and may distort the message. So sensitivity on the part of referees and attention to stylistic considerations on the part of prospective authors are required.

Journals owe it to their ever increasing 'foreign' readership to publish good English. In-house processes ought to be in place to correct spelling and grammar mistakes made by 'foreign' authors and to defend good surgical prose against infiltration by jargon.

Chapter 9

Essential

statistics

G. D. Murray

Professor of Medical Statistics and
Head of Public Health Sciences
Department of Community Health Sciences
University of Edinburgh
Edinburgh, UK

Introduction

The need to prepare a manuscript reporting research findings is often the stimulus for a researcher to start thinking about the statistical aspects of their work. Indeed, for many would-be authors it is the receipt of the first rejection letter which initiates statistical thinking. Certainly when investigators seek statistical advice it is often at this late stage, by which time the role of the statistician becomes that of a salvage contractor. The single most important message which any reader should take from this chapter is that statistics does not provide the 'quick fix' which turns raw data into an elegant publication. Rather, statistical thinking should permeate the entire research process, from the precise formulation of a research question through the choice of an appropriate study design, the drafting of the research protocol, grant application and ethics submission, the logistical planning and conduct of the study, the handling of any changes to and deviations from the protocol, to the final stages of analysis, presentation and interpretation of the results.

A great deal of clinical research is undertaken by individuals with inadequate training or supervision in research methods. Altman's 1994 *BMJ* leading article 'The scandal of poor medical research' [1] makes this point forcibly, as do a large number of articles which have reviewed the statistical aspects of the medical literature [2-7]. The clear consensus of over 150 such review articles is that around 50% of published articles contain clear statistical errors. Although this problem is far from being resolved, it is increasingly being acknowledged. Major grant awarding bodies, regional and local research ethics committees, and journals are increasingly making use of statistical referees in their review processes.

Another key point to grasp is that errors in the analysis, presentation and interpretation of results can easily be rectified. What cannot be resolved are errors in the design or conduct of a study. This emphasises again how important it is to seek statistical advice at the very outset of a research project, when there is still the potential to fine tune the research question and to match the study design and sample size to that question. The study should then have the potential to provide a meaningful answer.

Taking this idea of following through a carefully constructed research question, it is an excellent discipline to sketch out a draft of the final paper at the stage that the study is being designed. It should be feasible to write the introduction, setting the research question in context, at this stage. The methods, including the justification for the sample size, should also be decided *a priori*. Moreover, it should also be possible to decide on the content of the tables and figures. Typically a study will need to be reduced to three or four tables and a couple of figures. If it is not clear at the design stage what data are going to be presented, then the research question is not sufficiently well defined. As well as focusing the mind, this approach is enormously useful in rationalising data collection. There is a strong tendency to try to measure everything that can be measured, producing large quantities of data that are never even analysed. This is wasteful and dilutes the quality of all of the data which are collected, including those data which actually matter.

Resources

Fortunately there is a wide range of resources which can provide guidance on the statistical aspects of medical research. Altman [8], Bland [9] and Campbell and Machin [10] have written excellent introductory texts, and a recent book by Campbell [11] covers some more advanced topics (logistic regression; survival analysis; random effects models) at an introductory level. A recent second edition of 'Statistics with Confidence' [12] by Altman *et al* explains the principles which support the strong preference of statisticians to use confidence intervals to present and interpret the results of a statistical analysis rather than relying upon p-values. The book also includes a Windows-based computer programme which can calculate confidence intervals for a wide range of standard analyses.

A number of journals provide clear statistical advice for their authors. The *BMJ* is particularly prominent in this area and their website (www.bmj.com) provides detailed guidance, including a series of checklists. The checklists are actually for the use of reviewers, but they provide an excellent *aide-mémoire* for authors as well, highlighting the points that referees will expect to have been addressed.

In the area of randomised clinical trials there is a set of widely accepted guidelines for how the design, conduct, analysis and interpretation of a trial should be reported. These 'CONSORT' guidelines have recently been updated [13] (see Appendix III), and many journals require their authors to adhere to the CONSORT guidelines. There is a similar set of guidelines for reporting meta-analyses (QUOROM [14], see Appendix II), although these guidelines have not as yet been adopted as widely as the CONSORT guidelines.

The fundamental principle underlying CONSORT is the idea of full disclosure. This can in fact be usefully extended to all scientific reporting. Research in the real world is never straightforward, and it is always preferable to be open in discussing problems and flaws in one's work, rather than waiting for them to be highlighted by referees [15] or in correspondence columns.

Detailed Guidance

In two linked papers in the *British Journal of Surgery* [16, 17] I discussed in general the statistical aspects of research methodology and also gave a set of relatively proscriptive guidelines for prospective authors. I would refer the reader to these for more detail and in the remainder of this chapter will expand upon some of the issues raised earlier and attempt to give some detailed advice.

Introduction / Methods

It is essential to set out clearly the purpose of the study, and, in particular, the precise research question must be specified. The choice of the study design needs to be discussed in the context of the research question. If the study is interventional, then ideally the design should be a randomised trial. If a weaker design is chosen, then this needs to be justified. Whatever the choice of study design, it is crucial to explain the way in which the sample size was determined. This should be on the basis of a statistical power calculation, which not only ensures that the study will have the potential to give a clear and robust answer to the primary research question, but also serves to flag unambiguously what is being taken as the primary outcome measure, and what effect size is to be regarded as being clinically relevant. This raises a point which is crucial in the eventual analysis and interpretation of the results, namely that the research question should always be posed in terms of trying to quantify the effect of an intervention or the strength of an association. For example, do not ask whether a new protocol for antibiotic prophylaxis will reduce the incidence of post-operative infection, but rather try to estimate the magnitude of the reduction. (This is not to prejudge that the intervention is effective, as the results might well be consistent with no reduction).

It is also crucial to set out what one might call the philosophical basis of the study and this comes down to a dichotomy. Are you performing a scientific experiment under highly artificial laboratory conditions, trying to get an insight into underlying mechanisms, or are you trying to answer a question in the real but messy world of clinical medicine. With the former explanatory approach you are generally trying to assess whether an intervention has the potential to be useful, whereas with the latter pragmatic approach you are asking whether such potential can be realised [16]. This distinction has a profound effect on how the study should be designed and conducted, and also determines the extent to which the findings may be generalised.

The methods section should set out the approach to the statistical analysis. Routine methods do not need to be described in detail, but it can be useful to discuss, for example, whether parametric or non-parametric methods will be adopted. Any non-standard or advanced methods should be justified and explained. It can also be helpful to reference the statistical package used for such analyses, although this is unnecessary for routine analyses. If performing a multivariate analysis, such as an adjusted comparison based on a logistic or a Cox regression, it is far more important to describe the strategy used to select covariates for the model than it is to report which computer package was used.

For a randomised clinical trial, the CONSORT guidelines [13] set out which details should be reported. It is particularly important to describe the mechanisms used to generate the treatment allocations, and to keep each allocation blind until the corresponding patient has been recruited into the trial.

Data Presentation

For data presentation, whether by graph or numerical summaries, the guiding principle should again be transparency. It should almost always be possible to present the results of a surgical study in such a way that the interpretation is self-evident. The formal statistical analysis is still vital to give objective confirmation of the subjective impression, but its role is supportive rather than central. Whenever possible a graph should show the actual data points rather than simply presenting some summary measure together with a possibly ill-specified 'error bar'. When the sample size is too large to show individual data points then a summary such as a box-and-whisker plot is invaluable in showing the 'shape' of a distribution, which in turn allows the reader to judge whether the formal statistical analysis is appropriate. Summary statistics must also reflect the shape of the distributions. For example, the mean and the standard deviation are only useful summaries when the data follow the familiar bell-shaped normal distribution. If the data are skewed then it is generally more appropriate to present the median and quartiles (which also form the basis of the box-and-whisker plot).

Data Analysis

The results section will generally start with a description of the study population, or, for a comparative study, a baseline comparison of the different groups. If the study is a randomised trial then the common practice of performing formal statistical comparisons of the groups at baseline is inappropriate. All that a statistical test does is to assess whether any observed difference might possibly have arisen by chance. With a randomised trial it is known that any observed baseline imbalance has arisen by chance (unless there could be some improper subversion of the randomisation process) and so there is no point testing this hypothesis. This is not to say that baseline imbalances are unimportant, but what matters is whether the imbalance is in a factor which is strongly related to the primary outcome variable. A modest imbalance in an important covariate which is far from being statistically significant could have a major impact on the interpretation of the results, whereas a substantial difference which is highly statistically significant could be totally irrelevant if it occurs in a variable which is only weakly associated with the primary outcome variable. The impact of such imbalances needs to be explored via adjusted analyses. Baseline comparisons are at best unnecessary and at worst highly misleading [18].

The primary analysis should relate directly to the research question, which will also be reflected in the *a priori* power calculation. The result of this analysis should almost always consist of an estimate of the parameter of interest (such as the percent reduction in the incidence of post-operative infection) along with its corresponding 95% confidence interval. It can also be useful to quote the corresponding p-value, but this should be in addition to the confidence interval rather than in place of it.

It is always tempting and often appropriate to back up the primary analysis with a series of secondary analyses, relating for example to secondary outcome variables or to subgroup analyses. It is useful to pre-specify a small number of such analyses in the study protocol, and it should be explicit in the results section whether particular secondary results were pre-specified or data-driven. There is nothing inherently wrong with data-driven analyses provided you follow the principle of transparency and make it utterly explicit that there has been no 'data dredging'. All too often one sees manuscripts where one data-driven comparison is highlighted in the abstract as being statistically significant, when this result is almost certainly a spurious false positive and very distant from the primary question. The abstract must focus on the primary question.

Interpretation

The interpretation must bring together the primary research question, the clinically relevant difference (as identified in the power calculation) and the 95% confidence interval for this difference. Almost always one sets out to show evidence of a treatment effect or of an association. If the confidence interval for the relevant difference excludes the value of zero then it is established that there is a difference. The lower end of the confidence interval indicates whether it has been established that there is a clinically relevant difference. For example, if against a control rate of post-operative infection of 8% one had a confidence interval for the reduction of 3% to 7% then this is both statistically and clinically significant. In other words, the reduction is at least 3%, which by any criterion is of clinical relevance. If, however, the confidence interval had been 0.1% to 5% then again this result would be statistically significant (since the interval does not include the value of zero). However, the data are consistent with a reduction as low as 0.1% and so it cannot be claimed to have established for certain that there is a treatment benefit which is clinically relevant.

There is even more scope for misinterpreting a 'non-significant' result. Here the confidence interval includes the value of zero, and so the results are consistent with no effect. If the power calculation has been stringent then the confidence interval will be narrow, and any clinically relevant difference will have been excluded. This would be a 'strong negative' finding which would establish the equivalence of the groups in terms of the primary outcome measure. If, however, the power calculation was rather liberal, then the confidence interval will be wide and include some values which are of clear clinical relevance. Such a study gives a 'weak negative' which is essentially uninformative.

It is crucial that what is taken as a clinically relevant difference is established *a priori*, as it plays a crucial role in the interpretation of the results. This is illustrated very clearly in a case of research misconduct highlighted recently in the *BMJ* [15, 19]. The study was a randomised controlled trial of foetal heart monitoring in spontaneous uncomplicated labour, with the primary outcome measure being the rate of umbilical arterial metabolic acidosis. In the original study protocol the clinically relevant difference was stated as being 3%. As the trial progressed there were various problems with patient recruitment (as is so often the case) and the power calculation was revised to take 4% as the smallest clinically relevant difference. The confidence interval calculated at the end of the trial was -2.3% to 3.5%. This is a 'negative' result which does not exclude the originally stated clinically relevant difference of 3%. According to the original protocol the trial is, therefore, uninformative but the confidence interval does exclude the reinterpreted minimum clinically relevant difference of 4%. The study suddenly becomes a strong negative finding which establishes the equivalence of the two interventions in terms of the rates of metabolic acidosis. Such mid-course adjustments are very common in clinical trials, but where the authors erred was that they did not report the original power calculation but rather reported the final power calculation as if it had been what was specified in the original study protocol. This example shows how the power calculation has a profound impact on how the results are interpreted, and illustrates yet again that full disclosure is crucial.

Conclusion

Statistical thinking is not always straightforward, but it is inseparable from the research process. All authors of medical research should strive to get to grips with the basic principles, using some of the excellent resources described above, and should also seek out statistical advice at an early stage. Although the ideas can be subtle, there is no reason why a paper reporting the results of a well-designed study should be difficult to follow. Indeed it is only when inadequate thought has been given during the design phase that the reporting can become tortuous. Simplicity and transparency are the prerequisites for good scientific writing.

References

1   Altman DG. The scandal of poor medical research. *BMJ* 1994; 308: 283-284.

2   Andersen B. *Methodological Errors in Medical Research. An Incomplete Catalogue.* Blackwell, Oxford, 1990.

3   Pocock SJ, Hughes MD, Lee RJ. Statistical problems in the reporting of clinical trials. A survey of three medical journals. *New England Journal of Medicine* 1987; 317: 426-432.

4   Murray GD. The task of a statistical referee. *British Journal of Surgery* 1988; 75: 664-667.

5   Gore SM, Jones IG, Rytter EC. Misuse of statistical methods: critical assessment of articles in BMJ from January to March 1976. *BMJ* 1977; i: 85-87.

6   Smith DG, Clemens J, Crede W, et al. Impact of multiple comparisons in randomised clinical trials. *American Journal of Medicine* 1987; 83: 545-550.

7   Murray GD. Promoting good research practice. *Statistical Methods in Medical Research* 2000; 9: 17-24.

8   Altman DG. *Practical Statistics for Medical Research.* Chapman and Hall, London, 1991.

9   Bland M. *An Introduction to Medical Statistics*, 2nd Edition. Oxford Medical Publication, Oxford, 1995.

10   Campbell MJ, Machin D. *Medical Statistics: A Commonsense Approach*, 3rd Edition. Wiley, Chichester, 1999.

11 Campbell MJ. *Statistics at Square Two*. BMJ Books, London, 2001.

12 Altman DG, Machin D, Bryant TN, Gardner MJ. *Statistics with Confidence*, 2nd Edition. BMJ Books, London, 2000.

13 Moher D, Schulz KF, Altman DG, for the CONSORT Group. The CONSORT statement: revised recommendations for improving the quality of reports of parallel-group randomised trials. *Lancet* 2001; 357: 1191-1194.

14 Moher D, Cook DJ, Eastwood S, et al. Improving the quality of reports of meta-analyses of randomised controlled trials: the QUOROM statement. *Lancet* 1999; 354: 1896-1900.

15 Murray GD. Commentary: research governance must focus on research training. *BMJ* 2001; 322: 1461-1462.

16 Murray GD. Statistical aspects of research methodology. *British Journal of Surgery* 1991; 78: 777-781.

17 Murray GD. Statistical guidelines for The British Journal of Surgery. *British Journal of Surgery* 1991; 78: 782-784.

18 Altman DG, Dore CJ. Randomisation and baseline comparisons in clinical trials. *Lancet* 1990; 335: 149-153.

19 Mires G, Williams F, Howie P. Randomised controlled trial of cardiotocography versus Doppler auscultation of foetal heart at admission in labour in low risk obstetric population. *BMJ* 2001; 322: 1457-1461.

Commentary
by B. C. Reeves

Senior Lecturer in Epidemiology, Health Services Research Unit, London School of Hygiene and Tropical Medicine, London, UK

It is refreshing to have such a succinct summary of the essentials of statistics for clinical researchers. Rather than simply repeating the mantra about obtaining statistical advice at the start, Professor Murray illustrates the way in which statistical thinking throughout a study produces better research. He points out why this is true in fundamental aspects, such as the number of patients required for a study to be able to detect a clinically

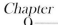
important effect, and more subtle ones, such as handling changes to and deviations from the original protocol.

There are many useful tips. Thinking about what will be the key results and how they will be laid out is one of the very best ways to clarify a research question and to decide which data really need to be collected. Errors in statistical analyses can be rectified but the study design and its conduct cannot. This is the most salient message in prompting researchers to seek advice before data collection starts rather than after it has finished.

The pressure to publish has become so great that researchers sometimes forget that clinical research is carried out to advance and inform health care. Research papers are used by others who may not be researchers themselves. The emphasis on the need for transparency in reporting research findings, and the way in which statistics help researchers to achieve this, is therefore especially welcome. The need to help users of research to understand the limitations of a study, rather than to disguise them from referees, should be a guiding principle. This point is highlighted by guidelines on reporting of research findings such as CONSORT.

Professor Murray's chapter is an excellent summary of these fundamental statistical aspects of surgical research - and certainly one to which I will direct those seeking guidance in the future.

Chapter 10

Writing about a surgical technique

A. Hirshberg

Associate Professor of Surgery

Michael E. DeBakey Department of Surgery

Baylor College of Medicine, Houston, Texas, U.S.A.

K. L. Mattox

Professor and Vice Chairman

Michael E. DeBakey Department of Surgery

Baylor College of Medicine, Houston, Texas, U.S.A.

&

Chief of Staff and Chief of Surgery

Ben Taub General Hospital, Houston, Texas, U.S.A.

Introduction

The written and graphical description of operative techniques is a unique feature of surgical literature that distinguishes it from publications in other medical fields. Surgical registrars or residents soon discover that a good atlas or operative textbook becomes an extremely valuable companion throughout their training. For many, this evolves into a lifelong fascination with technical surgical literature.

Surgeons read about operative techniques with much interest simply because the new technical knowledge is often directly applicable to patient care. Technical surgical writing does not follow the sequence of a scientific argument and may, therefore, be regarded by some as less prestigious than 'scientific' writing. It is, indeed, often personal and informal, but it is also very popular and of great practical importance for the clinical surgeon.

Many major surgical journals carry a technical section where surgeons share operative experiences and insights in an informal and practical way. The *American Journal of Surgery* and *Journal of the American College of Surgeons* carry regular technical sections where innovative surgical techniques and 'tricks' that facilitate the approach to technical problems are described. Comprehensive technical sections feature prominently in *Diseases of the Colon and Rectum* and in *Digestive Surgery*, where both new and traditional techniques are discussed in detail. Descriptions of new techniques appear intermittently in *Surgery*. Other journals, such as the *British Journal of Surgery* and *Archives of Surgery*, publish technical articles only as formal papers.

There are three major types of technical publications in surgery:

- Description of an entire procedure (such as gastrectomy or hernia repair).

- Discussion of the key element of a procedure (such as fashioning a colostomy or performing a vascular anastomosis).

- Technical 'tricks of the trade' that facilitate or simplify the performance of a problematic step.

In this chapter we will discuss some of the common underlying principles of technical writing and then briefly address each of the three types of technical publication.

General principles

Technical writing is typically the domain of the experienced author. For a technical article or chapter to be useful and publishable a critical mass of experience in both operative surgery and surgical writing is an obvious prerequisite.

When preparing to describe an operative technique, keep in mind that some readers are very likely to attempt the described technique in the operating room soon after publication. The author must be absolutely certain that the proposed technique actually works and is safe and sound.

The aim of the technical publication is to create in the reader's mind a clear and unambiguous mental picture of the procedure. This can best be accomplished by following a logical sequence, whereby each procedure is described as a series of discrete consecutive steps. For example, the generic steps of most operations are: access, exposure, exploration, resection, reconstruction and closure. Depending on the level of detail required for a specific description, each step can be further subdivided into several smaller steps.

The intelligent reader, however, expects much more than generic information from a technical publication. The reader expects to find insight and advice on how to actually apply the technique in the real world. This insight is usually provided by focusing on key maneuvers and major pitfalls.

A key maneuver is the single most important technical act during each operative step. For example, the key maneuver in dissecting the hilum of the gallbladder during an open cholecystectomy is identifying the junction of the cystic duct and common bile duct. In laparoscopic cholecystectomy, it is indentification of the junction of the gallbladder and the cystic duct. The key maneuver in exposing the carotid artery is division of the facial vein, and during dissection of the common femoral artery it is identification and looping of the deep femoral artery.

A major pitfall is a 'trap' that awaits the inexperienced during each operative step. During incision for an open appendectomy, a classical pitfall is placing the incision too medial. In preparing for a laparotomy for trauma a major pitfall is failure to include the chest and groins in the potential operative field.

The concept of the key maneuver and major pitfall is important because it allows a surgeon to transfer to others, by way of the printed word, 'inside knowledge' learned from experience. It is indeed this kind of insight that distinguishes the masterful description from a mere re-iteration of trivial technical detail. Professor Hugh Dudley, for example, has always provided this critical insight in his descriptions of operative procedures, including the most common difficulties and how to deal with them [1].

The artwork

A good technical description must be supported by effective illustrations that clearly enable the reader to grasp the essence of a critical step or technical refinement. This artwork may well be the most useful part of the article.

Converging an operative sequence into a single illustration is far from simple and much like trying to capture the essence of a video clip in one photograph. The writer must, therefore, run the operative sequence in his or her mind and carefully decide how to construct the illustration so it best serves its purpose. Photographs are an option, but usually fail to convey the full message and are therefore less popular.

The next step is enlisting the help of a professional medical illustrator. A good illustrator can work from a rough sketch or a photograph, but will usually work more effectively given a concrete example of an analogous situation from an operative atlas or anatomy book. A good collaboration between the author and the illustrator regarding the purpose of the illustration, and several iterations of the draft with close attention to detail will usually produce an illustration that is useful and visually appealing. The illustration does not have to be anatomically precise - it has to convey a message. Anatomical precision is thus often sacrificed in order to emphasize an important technical point or principle.

The full procedure

A chapter in a surgical atlas or textbook of operative surgery is the typical platform for this type of description. The intended audience is very broad so the description must be comprehensive and detailed and usually supported by several illustrations.

One feature that turns an operative description into a true 'pearl' is the inclusion of strategic and tactical considerations. The description should include not only the mechanics of the operative steps but also what is going on in the surgeon's mind as the procedure is performed. Strategy is the broad consideration of goals, alternatives and limitations of the procedure, while tactics are adjustments of a technique to specific conditions in the operative field. For example, the decision to employ temporary 'damage control' techniques during a laparotomy for trauma is a strategic decision, while the decision to perform a subtotal cholecystectomy is a tactical one.

The new technique

Before deciding to write up a novel operative technique, search the literature. It is not uncommon to find that a similar (or better) technique has already been described. Such descriptions sometimes predate electronic library databases so a search through older atlases in the historical section of a library may be very rewarding.

New techniques are typically published in the technical sections of surgical journals. The author can therefore assume that the audience consists of practicing surgeons familiar with the anatomy and the general conduct of the procedure. The description can focus on the novel approach itself and include a brief discussion of the advantages and disadvantages of the proposed new technique.

The 'useful trick'

When written well, these 'nuggets of practical wisdom' derived from the experience of others are a delight to read. They are, by nature, very brief communications, where clarity of description is the most important aspect. The technical refinement or trick should be described within the context of the procedure it is intended to facilitate, but there is no need to describe the entire procedure. For example, a description of a technique to facilitate division of the mesentery during bowel resection should not include a detailed account of the bowel resection itself. A single effective illustration, often schematic and simple, is extremely valuable in imparting the essence of the proposed refinement to the reader.

Summary

Technical writing in surgery is a special challenge that requires a methodical and well planned approach. The reader of a technical note or chapter expects not only a clear description of the mechanical side but, even more importantly, the methodical discussion of intra-operative considerations, strategies and tactics.

A technical description should follow a logical sequence, address potential traps and pitfalls, and be supported by effective graphical material. Despite the informal 'non-scientific' nature, technical publications are extremely valuable additions to the surgical knowledge base.

References

1   Dudley HAF. Chapter 33: Acute Appendicitis. In: Dudley HAF (ed): *Hamilton Bailey's Emergency Surgery*. 11th Ed. 1986, Bristol, John Wright & Sons, pp 336 - 345.

Commentary
by A. Darzi
Professor of Surgery, St. Mary's Hospital, London, UK

The authors have acknowledged the importance of surgical technique writing and emphasised the popularity of this over the last decade with the introduction of minimally invasive surgery. Most major scientific surgical journals do now have sections dealing with entire procedures, as highlighted by the author, or 'tricks of the trade'.

Surgery is one of the few technical specialities that lends itself to the process of technical mapping in which each step of a procedure can be described with good illustrations to highlight the logical sequence. Although the authors are using main themes such as access, exposure, exploration, resection, reconstruction and closure; each individual aspect of these could be further mapped to help explain the operative procedure in a written format.

One point which is gaining popularity is the impact of technology and multimedia in the description of surgical technique in the future. There are one or two examples of highly popular websites through which an operative procedure is mapped by text and associated clips of video. With band width becoming cheaper and much more available, it is anticipated that the description of surgical techniques and new procedures would probably be best described with the integration of text, animation, video clips and even possibly virtual reconstruction of organs. These would significantly enhance the reader's perception of the steps of an operative procedure.

Chapter 11

The final product

J. A. Murie

Consultant Vascular Surgeon

&

Honorary Senior Lecturer

Royal Infirmary of Edinburgh

Edinburgh, UK

The completed manuscript - The Final Product - lies in front of you on your desk. What happens next? Do not be tempted to cram it rashly into an envelope and bear it with speed to the nearest post box. A moment's quiet contemplation at this point may avoid needless delay and embarrassment at a later stage when obvious, simple faults are uncovered by referees and editors.

Preparation of manuscripts

You will probably have had some idea of the journal to which your work might be sent for some time. Once a final selection has been made, sit down with the manuscript and the appropriate Instructions to Authors. These Instructions can be found in each issue of many journals and, if not, you will be pointed to a relevant issue or website by the Editorial Office of the publication concerned. Check your work carefully against the Instructions. It is surprising how many manuscripts have glaring, yet simple defects. These may result in a return of your work for revision even before peer review, typically entailing a delay of two weeks or more.

Authors should also consider the matter of English language spelling (English style or American style) and tailor their efforts appropriately. This should be straightforward in the present computerised era in which word processing spell-checkers are widely available for both styles. The point is especially relevant if submission is being made to a journal of second choice that uses spelling of a style different from that of the first choice publication. Journals can, of course, revise the spelling in-house and will rarely require authors to re-draft on this count alone, but sending a manuscript in the 'wrong' style is lax at best and discourteous at worse.

Should your efforts fail to gain editorial approval at the journal of your first choice, you may select a second journal. Be particularly careful to study the ethos and style of this second choice in case it differs from that of your first selection. Ensure that your manuscript

is appropriately presented and if necessary alter it appropriately. The receipt of work in the style of journal A by the editors of (second choice) journal B is not likely to enhance your chances of making a good impression. Deep down all editors know that their journal is not always the 'first choice', but superficially it is a fiction that they like to maintain and you should collude with them in this.

Authorship

Agreement on authorship should have occurred at a very early stage in your research [1]. Still, this is your last chance to consider this serious matter before your work leaves for the public domain. The award of authorship should be given only to those making a substantial contribution to conception, design, analysis and writing of the study, or collection of data [2]. For those making lesser contributions it may be that an acknowledgement is more appropriate. If your author total seems excessive, it is probable that editors will question the roles played by these individuals; common sense and frankness at the pre-submission stage is better than embarrassment later. Be especially cautious if including more than six putative authors and consider justification for seven or more authors in your letter of submission.

All authors are generally invited to sign a letter of submission to accompany the manuscript. This is an important step which should not be regarded lightly. By signing such a letter you are usually attesting to several matters. First, you will be stating that the work has not previously been accepted for publication or published elsewhere, or that is has been simultaneously submitted elsewhere. If an abstract of the work and a foreign language version have been published previously these must be declared fully in your letter of submission. Second, you will probably be agreeing formally that you have no potential or actual political or financial interest in the material submitted or, if you do, stating explicitly what this might be. It is obvious that all authors must study the manuscript with care before its submission. To sign a letter of submission without so doing is negligent and severe retribution has been known to follow an improper signature. In summary, treat your professional signature with the respect it deserves.

In a better world the last paragraph would have been written solely for the tyro. Sadly, in the actual world one must make a plea for heads of departments and other senior authors to reflect on its substance. The *BJS*, for example, receives a small yet regular supply of manuscripts which are so deeply flawed (in substance and/or presentation) that the editors cannot believe the senior authors have read them. Still, these papers are accompanied by a letter of submission that has been signed by all authors. Are <u>you</u> guilty?

Peer review and the editor's decision

Your paper will be assessed by the editor, usually with the help of one or more referees. Referees are generally established experts who themselves have a track record in publishing learned articles and who are well regarded by the journal. A decision may be made to reject your work; the rejected article will be discussed later in this book and no further comment is made here. On the other hand, the editor may decide to accept your paper without revision, but this is a very rare event indeed. Most papers achieve eventual acceptance only after revision in the light of the referees' and editor's comments.

If you are offered the opportunity to re-submit after revision, you should deal with all the points made and state in a covering letter what exactly has been done. Editors and referees are not infallible. Very occasionally a point is made that is erroneous or unreasonable. In such circumstances your covering letter must state clearly why you cannot or will not make the requested changes. You must be confident in your argument, however, as professional arrogance in discounting a reasonable request is a certain way of ensuring rejection of your work. In general, the points raised by journal referees are invaluable in enhancing the quality of the finished product. It often surprises the editors of *BJS* how much time is lost during the revision stage. It is desirable to proceed quickly with recasting your manuscript to ensure it does not become dated. Enlightened self interest also demands rapid attention to your paper because you cannot claim it as being 'in press', only 'in preparation' - a far less convincing situation if you wish to cite the work in a curriculum vitae or bibliography.

Page proofs

After acceptance, you will receive page proofs of your paper before its eventual publication. These show the layout of your text and illustrations, and are sent to authors for careful checking; again, delay is to be avoided. Although the editors and internal proof readers will also scrutinise the work at this stage, input from authors is essential. You must check that what you want to say has come out clearly and that no alteration (by you or by the editors) has inadvertently distorted your original message. Rarely, mistakes occur, and while these can always be corrected by an erratum (journal's error) or a corrigendum (author's error) in a later issue of the journal, this is obviously undesirable. Others who access your article in the future may not be aware of the erratum or corrigendum, which inevitably appears in a separate issue of the publication concerned.

If proper care has been taken at manuscript stage, the number and size of changes at proof stage should be minimal. Proofs do not lend themselves to major alterations and are not intended for that purpose.

Copyright

In medical publishing it is widespread practice for a journal (or book) publisher to request that you assign copyright to the publisher. In certain circumstances a writer might wish to retain copyright; this can sometimes be accommodated if there is a good reason for the request and the editors greatly desire to publish the text in question.

The usual circumstance is when an author is part of an organization (a medical defence union for instance) that routinely retains copyright for any professional text written by its staff. In general, however, copyright passes to the journal and, at least so far, this has rarely caused difficulty. Requests to reproduce your work (or part of it) are not unreasonably withheld by any of the established medical publishing houses. With the obvious exception of deliberate dual publication of your article, you will be free to use extracts of your text and illustrations in future work, should you feel this to be desirable. You should make the necessary and due acknowledgement of the source.

There is one situation, however, in which some editors would allow deliberate dual publication and this relates to a re-print of a paper in a second language (generally the native language of the authors). This usually occurs in a small domestic journal after first exposure in English in a mainstream publication. Those who hold this view defend the practice on the grounds that not every reader understands English and it is the work of editors to help in the dissemination of knowledge. On the other hand, if carried to an extreme, every paper could appear in several languages in several journals and it is no one's interest to expand publication needlessly. Publication of a paper in more than one language must be handled sensitively and every case dealt with on its own merits. It should only be allowed on rare occasions when the case for extended dissemination of information is unarguable. Permission must be sought by the second publisher from those who hold the copyright; the former must highlight the fact that the paper is a reproduction and give a clear reference of the original source. Guidance on this issue can also be found in the Vancouver Guidelines.

Letters to the editor

Many journals have correspondence pages and *BJS* is one such journal. Much correspondence relates to work that has recently been published in the journal and it is common practice for an editor to send any letter received about a paper to that paper's corresponding author. In this way the authors should be able to answer questions about their work raised by readers and to rebut criticism. A healthy correspondence section is the mark of a vibrant, successful journal. Editors will welcome your thoughtful and (again) speedy response to letters they have received.

Electronic publishing

Before concluding, a few thoughts on electronic publication seem apposite in the current age. It is certain that the 'final product' in your chosen paper journal will eventually find its way on to the internet; for instance, *BJS* is published both on paper and electronically. In these circumstances the electronic version is simply a copy of the paper product. Electronic publication, however, lends itself to a new form of publication activity, that is 'pre-publishing'. This may take the form of placing your text on a web site as soon as it is accepted by journal editors and without final editorial alteration. It may even take the form of web site placement before acceptance, even before peer review; indeed the internet allows publication without peer review and even despite rejection by hitherto well regarded filtering mechanisms (otherwise known as journal editors). In these circumstances your product will, to a greater or lesser extent, be unchanged by any editorial hand. Your true writing and presentational abilities will lie naked for all to see. Maybe the ease of electronic publication will produce a spate of rapidly, casually and (perhaps) carelessly written articles. The more mature author will, however, reflect on the nature of net publication and take even greater care than before.

Conclusion

The true 'final product' is, of course, your article published inside the pages of a prestigious journal. To reach this stage regularly you must work with speed and with care. Remember also that your text and letters are being sent into the public domain. Sign only that which you are confident about and encourage in your colleagues a similar degree of probity when dealing with editors and their publishers.

References

1   Guidelines on good publication practice. Committee on Publication Ethics. *Br J Surg* 2000; 87: 135.

2   Guidelines on good publication practice. Committee on Publication Ethics. *Br J Surg* 2000; 87: 265.

Commentary
by A. E. Young
Consultant Surgeon, St. Thomas' Hospital, London, UK

'The editor's decision is final' is an oft-quoted truth that hopeful authors ignore at their peril. By and large editors are good natured and charitable creatures who but for the constraints of space would publish much more of what is submitted to them. The editor is however the nub of the journal publishing business. Pressures can sometimes make editors tetchy so it behoves the author to help as much as possible and not to cause irritation. Adherence to all the advice in this chapter will go a long way to achieving that end.

John Murie's crucial message is to pause and reflect before submitting your final product. To you it is the gratifying distillation of much hard work of which you are proud; or which you wish simply to get behind you, preferably by way of an entry on your c.v. Your confidence in the paper's value, accuracy and readability, however, may be misplaced. Pause and reflect. What may seem clear to you who lived with the paper for so long and revised it so often may be opaque to a naïve reader; so get a colleague who is not involved in the project to read it through. Ask specifically for comments on the overall structure of the paper, its presentation and readability. If you aren't specific about this you will probably find that the text simply comes back altered to match the reader's own grammatical prejudices. Also ask about the illustrations and figures. Do they make sense, particularly photographs? These will be smaller and less defined when printed. A good trick is to give your colleague the illustrations photocopied at a quarter A4 size. If he can still work out what they show then submit them but expect the majority of photomicrographs and operative photos to end up in the bin.

Lastly, when you actually submit you paper make sure it is clean and tidy, the pages and illustrations numbered. Then put it out of your mind for the editor is a busy person as are his referees; a decision on your paper will always take longer than your impatience predicts.

Chapter 12

*What an editor
wants or expects
from authors*

C. H. Organ, Jr.

Professor and Chairman

Department of Surgery

University of California-San Francisco

Oakland, California

U.S.A.

In an ideal world the editor finds gratification in reviewing the work of authors who demonstrate an appreciation for the responsibility and obligations of authorship with its professional and personal rewards. It is mutually beneficial to the editor and author if the latter is familiar with the guidelines initially issued by the International Conference of Medical Journal Editors in 1985 [1] and the uniform requirements for manuscripts submitted to biomedical journals issued in 1997 [2]. We are what we write. The editor expects the author, prior to submitting a manuscript, to have read the journal's instructions for authors and to have implemented these instructions with precision and honesty.

Detailed attention should be directed to copyright requirements, the accuracy of references, a clear definition of author responsibility, titles, illustrations, legends, and tables. The editor expects the author to be familiar with the elements of informed consent, full financial disclosure, protection of patient privacy, animal experiment guidelines, Institutional Review Board requirements, photographic consent, and statistical review where and when appropriate. Compliance with these details avoids format changes, publication delay, unnecessary correspondence and taxation of the editor's patience. If everything is present in a manuscript, it facilitates entering data into a computerized typing system for processing and an early decision.

Fundamental to what editors want and expect from authors is embodied in the structured abstract: a clearly stated hypothesis, study design, the setting, intervention studies, outcome measures, results, and conclusions justified by the data. Data extraction for quality and validity is the editorial prerequisite which leads to quantitative and qualitative results. 'In God we trust, but everyone else must have data.'

Authors should be aware of specific details that attract the attention of the editor when reviewing manuscripts. The editor expects authors to avoid submitting manuscripts on highly specialized topics that are not of fundamental interest to the journal's readership. The author is expected to have participated sufficiently in the work to take full responsibility for its content. Although 'substantial contribution' has not been clearly defined and is a work in progress, editors want authors to be involved in one or more of the following areas:

◆ conception, design, analysis, and interpretation of the data;

◆ drafting the manuscript or revising it critically for content; and

◆ approving the published version of the manuscript [3].

An excessive number of authors (more than age) creates the question of complimentary authorship.

Recent proposals to replace the current system of authorship with unambiguous credits for specific contributions should be encouraged. This grouping of all authors collectively as 'authors' is neither tenable nor responsible. Collaborative interdisciplinary research has encouraged inflated authorship and in so doing has likewise disseminated responsibility. The editor expects authors to be sensitive to the current trends and responsibilities of authorship inflation.

An increasing number of bibliometric studies confirm that as many as 30% of published articles may be classified as duplication of previously published articles (i.e. redundant publication, salamization). Editors are sensitive and usually responsive to both duplication and duplicity. Editors expect authors to obey the simple rule: 'if it has been in print, and especially if it has been peer reviewed, it shouldn't be put in print again' [4]. In an era of electronic publishing and computers, authors should expect that editors may generate a computerized database of previous and current work for comparison. Editors of different journals communicate with each other in a collaborative way to detect and exclude duplication.

Edward G. Huth has reminded us that 'wasteful publication includes dividing the results in a single study into two or more papers (salami-slice science)': republishing the same material in successive papers (which need not have identical forms and content) or in blending data from one study with additional data to extract another paper that would not make its way on the second set of data alone (meat extenders) [5]. Authors should be aware that editors look for and discourage serial publication.

What does the editor expect from the authors? Respect for the peer review process, prompt reply to inquiries from the editor, and full financial disclosure. The editor expects authors to understand the peer review system, its anonymity, and to realize that it is a slow, expensive, and time-consuming process. Full disclosure from the editor, peer reviewer and author lend credibility to the process. The authors should expect that their work will not be reviewed where a conflict of interest or the possibility of a biased review may enter the equation. Journal editors want, and look forward to reviewing, manuscripts of reasonable length (not words without end, amen). To investigate and track down certain elements of a manuscript, particularly if funded by the biomedical industrial complex, is not a profitable use of the editor's time. The editor expects adherence to sound grammatical structure. This includes the avoidance of slang, minimal abbreviations, the absence of dangling participles, split infinitives and parallelism. (See chapter 7, 'Advice on writing style').

Intellectual property is a legal term that results in the creative efforts of the mind (intellectual), which can be owned, possessed and subject to competing claims (property). Three legal doctrines govern intellectual property:

◆ copyright (the law protecting authorship and publication);

◆ patent (the law protecting invention and technology); and

◆ trademark (the law protecting words and symbols used to identify goods and services in the marketplace) [6].

The editor expects authors to respect all three.

Editors expect authors to understand that an accepted manuscript becomes the permanent property of the journal and may not be published without permission from the publisher. Editors prefer that authors minimize self-citations, unpublished data and personal communications.

Editors expect authors to realize that affiliation agreements with surgical societies do not guarantee publication even though they are reviewed and selected by a program committee for presentation. Although this is an initial review process, the editor and editorial board make the final decision. Presentation at a national meeting is based on a review of the abstract, not the complete manuscript. The editor would hope each author realizes that the peer review process is currently the best we have to offer and that manuscripts are usually improved by this process. The editor expects authors to avoid overall indictments and subjective comments. Disagreements (even debates) between the author, reviewer, and editor are healthy and usually result in an improved manuscript. The editor expects authors to refrain in their manuscript and/or responses to the editor from accusations, unkind remarks, and abusive language. We prefer to seek humour and comedy relief elsewhere.

The editor expects that the submission of a manuscript is an assurance from the author(s) to both the editor and readers that this is an original publication. Authors should understand the responsibilities of the editor and editorial board to produce a quality publication. The editor in turn believes that the submitted manuscript should provide an educational process for the reader, editor and author. Everyone must cooperate in producing information that improves the science of surgery and ultimately patient care. Editors expect authors to appreciate that clinical manuscripts will undergo the same rigid review as work in basic science. The editor expects authors to refrain from distribution of the manuscript prior to publication (publication by press conference) and to abide by the embargo policy of the journal [7]. The editor expects the author to appreciate that the submitted manuscript is a privileged communication.

Editors have an immense responsibility and expect authors to believe:

◆ that their manuscripts will be reviewed fairly and receive honest feedback;

◆ the editor to be an honest and objective adjudicator, and

◆ the editor to be equitable and prudent in the selection of reviewers.

Peer reviewers do not always concur, requiring the editor to make the final decision. These decisions have an element of subjectivity. We do our very best to make a well-informed, unbiased decision. The author is expected to understand that manuscript rejection is often multifactorial, based largely on editorial priorities, a restriction in the number of pages available, reader interest, etc. Editors expect authors to appreciate that editors do know how it feels to receive a rejection letter. Manuscript acceptance is an occasion for quiet celebration and satisfaction for both author and editor.

References

1   International Committee of Medical Journal Editors' Guidelines on Authorship. *Br Med J*. 1985; 291: 722.

2   International Committee of Medical Journal Editor's Uniform Requirements from Manuscripts Submitted to Biomedical Journals. *JAMA*. 1997; 277: 927-934.

3   American Medical Association Manual of Style: A Guide For Authors. 9th Edition. Williams & Wilkins. 1998. Page 100-123.

4   Kennedy D. *Academic Duty*. Harvard Press. Cambridge, Massachusetts. 1997. Page 195.

5   American Medical Association Manual of Style: A Guide For Authors. 9th Edition. Williams & Wilkins. 1998. Page 99.

6   American Medical Association Manual of Style: A Guide For Authors. 9th Edition. Williams & Wilkins. 1998. Page 112.

7   Butler D. 'Publication by press conference' under fire. *Nature* 1993; 366: 6.

Commentary
by A. L. Warshaw

W. Gerald Austen Professor of Surgery, Harvard Medical School and Surgeon-in-Chief, Massachusetts General Hospital, Boston, U.S.A.

Claude Organ is the first Editor under whom I served as an Editorial Board member before going on to help lead my own journal, Surgery. His succinct Editor's guide to authors reminds me how much I learned from him: his precepts are to be followed. To those principal tenets - originality of material and responsible authorship, I dare to add and emphasize three desirable qualities for the subject of a journal article: importance, utility, and interest.

The primary purposes of a publication should not be to publicize the authors, to serve as a vehicle for their academic promotion, or to give patronage to senior colleagues. Rather, the potential contribution should be measured by its educational content, whether new or synthesized, and its relevance to the science and practice of surgery. The composition should avoid the turgid and exploit the richness of language. Those for whom English is not a comfortable medium can greatly improve the chances of acceptance for their work, as well as the chances that it will be read, by fastidious attention to composition with the help of a skilled writer. The message of a well-written manuscript is more likely to be comprehended, incorporated, and remembered. Arguably the most important attributes of good medical writing, however, are focus, logical progression of argument, and conciseness (the KISS principle: keep it simple, son). Authors are well advised to avoid the temptation to compress into the manuscript every observation and alternative nuance found in a literature search. I believe that after content this is the key to effective communication of the central message.

Although all might not agree, there can be a place for colourful language as well as a little lighter fare to forestall wavering attention. Prestigious journals now feature non-medical 'art' photographs (the New England Journal of Medicine), case quizzes (Gastroenterology), historical trivia (Archives of Surgery), and entertaining vignettes (Surgery). These elements do not substitute for serious content of medical and scientific excellence, but they do add attraction.

Finally, we should acknowledge what authors should expect from Editors and the reviewers they solicit: knowledge and depth of the subject at hand, serious analysis of the submission, fairness and balance, absence of conflict of interest, openness to new ideas and willingness to perform timely reviews. Do remember that every reviewer will again be an author in need of good reviewers.

Chapter 13

How to write a chapter

A. Fingerhut

Chief of Service, Digestive Surgery

Centre Hospitalier Intercommunal, Poissy, France

&

Associate Professor of Surgery

Louisiana State University Medical School

New Orleans, LA, U.S.A.

What to do when asked to write a book chapter

To be asked to write a chapter for a book is indeed an honour: this means that you have been chosen by the editors as an 'expert' in the field and that they want you to be the source of information for that particular theme in their book.

With this in mind, you should try to answer the following questions: The first question to ask yourself is: 'Do I feel qualified to write this chapter?' If not, just say 'Thank you' and refer the editors to someone else. If you do feel that this is your topic, then the second question is: 'Do I have the time to do it well?' Think twice about the time needed to plunge into an in-depth review of the topic and to actually write the chapter. Make a careful assessment of your other commitments and beware of saying 'yes' and then 'auto-plagiarizing' one of your previous chapters. This will not go unnoticed, will not contribute positively to your reputation and will not help the editors. The third question is: 'Should I do it myself or should I include one or more co-authors?' Who should the co-author(s) be? Local politics may dictate that it be your boss: talk to him or her beforehand. He or she may or may not want to be on the list of authors. You may want to include a more junior author and the obvious advantage here would be that the junior will do the hard work of data collecting. They would be compensated by having their name in print and by seeing you work, learning how to do it for the future. Beware of letting the junior do the actual writing unless you really know how good the chapter will be: rewriting is often much more work than doing the actual writing oneself. Letting a mediocre chapter go by with your name on it is inviting disaster. Last, but not least, be sure that you know the qualifications and intentions of the editors and their publishers. Writing a chapter is a great deal of work: you do not want to do it in vain!

The problems

One of the most frustrating problems in writing a chapter for a book is the harmony that has to be struck to enable each chapter to find its place and be integrated into what would otherwise be a heterogeneous mix. Book production is often a long and complex undertaking and in order to be factual and up to date, the editorial timetable is often restricted. Even so, most chapters are to some extent outdated when they come to press. Many book chapters are for books that seem to multiply but, by and large, dwell on the same overall topics, e.g. 'Dupont's operative manual'. Your task is double: do not duplicate chapters that may be found in other books (especially if you are the 'expert' author of both!) and find a novel, original aspect to your topic. The last and probably the most difficult problem (usually the editors' job, not the writers') is to make sure that there is a common denominator in the thought and contents of the book as a whole. This means following the instructions dictated by the editors. Ensure that clear instructions and the strategy of the book come with the letter of invitation. Remember that each and every one of the participants in the composition of a book have their role: contributors, editors and publishers have to work in step to ensure the quality of the end product.

Follow the sample chapter

While the actual contents are usually up to the author, the points to be covered, the style, the structure and the limitations should be dictated by the editors. This is best done through the letter of invitation (which is usually short and very unhelpful) and through a sample chapter. This should be provided at the outset with detailed editors' instructions (which are usually a bit longer and more helpful). The sample chapter should ideally be an original manuscript (chapter), written by the editors themselves. Their ideas and style should be the guiding principles for your own chapter. This sample chapter will make your (the writer's) task easier and assist you in producing a draft close to its final version in the customary short time frame available.

Follow the overall outline

In order to keep in tune with the general line of thought and to integrate your chapter into the overall trend of the book, it is essential that the editors provide you (and all the authors) with as complete an outline of the entire book as possible. This will allow you and the other authors to identify those chapters which might be redundant or overlap with others. As for your contribution, it might be a good idea to ask the authors of the chapters which might overlap, for a copy of their outline in order to come to some form of agreement on who covers what and in which order.

Title, subtitle (and citations)

The title of a book chapter is generally very broad and is part of the general plan of chapters made up by the editors. The actual title and above all the contents are more malleable. Even though the editors usually provide you with a title, do not hesitate to modify it, while sticking to the overall plan and general idea of the book. The title itself should be short, but eye-catching. Often one sees a 'citation' under the title. Provide one only if the editors ask for it. A subtitle is often useful to explain what the chapter contains.

Contents

Once you know what the structure of your chapter should be, you should think not only about its content, but how to integrate it in the overall content of the book to attract and interest the readership. You should have a definition of your target audience before starting to compose the chapter. Is it a textbook with a pedagogic goal? Is it a chapter about a particular topic of interest for you to relate your personal ideas or expertise? Is it a chapter about your current field of clinical expertise or research? Are illustrations, figures and photographs necessary or advisable? Will they enhance the comprehension? How should they be integrated into the text and how do they highlight the text? If the editors have not provided you with this information, do not hesitate to ask for it.

Outline

The structure is best understood when you, as an author, are able to jot down the main points as a proper outline. If the outline seems straightforward and falls well into line with the general outline of the book, continue. If not, or if there is any doubt as to what the editors expect, your outline should be sent back to the editors very early in the process. In this way they will be able to give their approval and advice before you continue too far in the process.

How to say it

As stated by Lewerich and Gotze [1], 'Do not tell the readers what **you know** about the subject, tell them what **they should know** about it'. Remember that most chapters are not peer-reviewed with the same level of expertise or incisiveness, as peer-reviewed, original papers. This is not an excuse for sloppy or incomplete data gathering or writing. As said before, beware of the temptation to leave the writing to an inexperienced junior. All writing, even in book chapters, requires tutorial guidance, coloured with the wisdom and experience of the senior mentor.

Writing (putting it down on paper)

A book chapter differs somewhat from an original paper. You should use (preferentially) the present tense for verbs. The past tense may, however, be used when commenting on another contribution from which you have decided to provide the readership with some details. Avoid using all other tenses. Chapters like this present one make use of the imperative. This is ideal when the chapter, as this one, is meant to be a guide on how to do something, rather than being 'just' instructive.

Use sub-headings freely, but make sure that they follow a sequential, logical, stream of thought.

The introduction is of paramount importance. A poor or unattractive introduction will discourage the reader. It should be short and concise and tell the reader what will be found in the remaining part of the chapter.

The body of the chapter should be factual. The authors' personal experience can be included, but ideally this should be in the form of citations. Do not usurp the chapter for your personal techniques, unless asked specifically by the editors to do so. Being factual means being impartial, honest with yourself and the others, complete, as well as comprehensive. Avoid sentences such as 'as shown (or discussed) later'. Making generous references to other chapters of the book to avoid redundancies, however, is recommended. The sequence of ideas should be able to stand alone and this is why an outline is useful.

A brief word about the format: remember that most books are published in columns. Think about this when composing.

Last, as we are now in the electronic age, e-books are developing rapidly. Writing an 'e-chapter' should not differ much from writing traditional book chapters. Owing to their pedagogic aspect, as opposed to original research papers, most book chapters can be updated without much ado, and the electronic format is the ideal way to do it. Ask the editors if this is part of your contract with the book so that you can plan on this from the start as, depending on the renewal schedule, the enterprise may be time-consuming.

Limitations

Limitations include the number of pages and references and the number and type (colour) of illustrations and tables.

Strict limitations to the number of pages and the number and type of illustrations and tables is usually dictated by economy of space and to keep costs to a minimum. These limitations should be adhered to strictly (by the authors). While, in most cases, the number of pages can always be re-edited (by the editors), it is best to stay within the rules from the outset. The line of thought or the overall message might otherwise be misinterpreted or camouflaged when a third party makes corrections. If, however, you find it absolutely necessary to alter length or content, modifications can usually be negotiated with the editors or the publishers. This should be done as early as possible in the project.

References can either be cited in the text but, most often, they are not. A bibliography can be used to list the most interesting references. Check with the sample chapter and/or the instructions for the authors. Obviously, only the most pertinent and recent references should be used. Remember that a chapter of a book is usually going to be read at least 12 to 18 months after you finish writing it. If the references are not cited in the text, include only (a few of) the top original articles, and concentrate on review articles. If the book has a precise topic, you may be asked to give a list of references that figure in a specific, separate chapter, provided for the entire book.

Illustrations occasionally provide a problem. They should be professional. Some books include original drawings of the authors (e.g. Mastery of Surgery). The idea is in itself quite original: as the chapters are usually on surgical techniques and surgeons are often good artists, this usually works out well.

If you are not a good artist, however, it is often necessary to engage a professional artist. Usually this is under the responsibility and expense account of the authors of the chapter, not of the editors. On the other hand, some publishing houses provide the artists (Encyclopaedias). Colour illustrations, however, are apart, as they are often very expensive and rarely add much more than black and white illustrations. These should be kept to a strict minimum. The exception, of course, would be the results of a Colour Doppler examination or a pathological specimen on a slide and this should have been integrated into the overall book costs. Obviously, a chapter on interventional radiology or CT scans will contain many figures, but these are usually in black and white.

Tables fit well into most book chapters and, unlike illustrations, do not cost much. They should be modest in size, clear and lightly spaced. They should be explicit and able to be read separately so that the reader need not consult the text to understand them.

Conclusion

Writing a chapter for a book is an enlightening experience but requires professional know-how and expertise. To do a good job means adhering to what the editors and the publishing house expects of you. To do an excellent job means implicating your part into the book as a whole. The timetable is usually strict and should be respected with a minimum of delay.

References

1   Lewerich B, Götze D. 'What to do when you are asked to write a chapter' in *Surgical Research. Basic principles and clinical practice.* Third Edition, Springer, New York. Editors: H Tröidl, MF McKneally, DS Mulder, AS Wechsler, B McPeek, WO Spitzer. 1998 pp 127-9.

Commentary
by M. W. Büchler
Professor of Surgery, Chairman, Department of General Surgery, University of Heidelberg, Heidelberg, Germany

I am pleased to write a commentary on 'How to write a book chapter'. In itself this chapter refills the criteria that are formulated by the author, namely to be concise, instructive, well organized, with subtitles and the content triggered to the needs of the target audience. I can only add some aspects of interpretation of editors', authors' and readers' needs in such book chapters.

Novelty for each chapter versus day to day realism (auto plagiarism)

The person invited to produce a book chapter is usually the expert in the field and this leads to frequent invitations. The work may be a standard textbook or proceedings following a meeting or Festschrift but nearly always brings honour and or prestige to the author and institution. To decline requests for writing is unusual and an author may, therefore, accrue several commitments to produce similar or related chapters for different books. It is then difficult to produce an entirely novel or unique contribution for each book. An element of auto plagiarism may be allowed in this setting since the books are likely to be targeted for slightly different groups or may even be produced in differing languages. Editors and readers alike should see this auto plagiarism through appropriate citations and acknowledgements.

Many authors use the repeated invitations to write in the training of junior academics by asking them to produce the work in first draft. This manoeuvre must be cleared by the senior editor and publishers of the book. The junior surgeon is the first author but the senior academic <u>must</u> have significant input into the structure and content of the chapter.

Harmony versus individualism

One of the major problems of surgical books is the lack of harmony across the chapters. Repetitive information in chapters and different wording, style and objectives may all be found in varying degree. I would, therefore, agree with Abe Fingerhut's request for strict outlines provided by editors beforehand. Unfortunately such planning instructions are frequently not provided and to harmonize such books provides an almost impossible task.

The timetable as a wonderful adventure

Some reality is necessary on the part of editors and authors for submission deadlines. I think that 3 months over time is the maximum of flexibility that can usually be tolerated in a management schedule.

Rejecting an invitation

Books are frequently produced by expert friends but despite the friendship the decision for accepting the chapter must be based exclusively upon the author's qualification and availability (time). Such rules should not be violated and a rejection must be regarded as a business decision and accepted.

Conclusion

To write a book chapter is a demanding and honourable job and the guidance perfectly outlined in this chapter should be followed. Once in a while, but not always, an excellent book chapter will be produced.

Chapter 14

How to edit or write a book

M. Schein

Professor of Surgery

Cornell University Medical College

&

Bronx Lebanon Hospital, New York

U.S.A.

Of making many books there is no end...

Bible, Ecclesiastes, 12:12

You are an accomplished academic surgeon and a recognized expert in your field and a publisher proposes that you 'do' a book. You may be a rising star; having already published a number of original papers and a few chapters and now you want to decorate your curriculum vitae and your coffee table - with your own book. Alternatively, you may be practicing away from the towers of academia but you have that great original idea nestling in your literary mind which you believe deserves a book. Whatever is your declared motivation for wanting to 'do' a book you must admit that the reason resides within your ego. This chapter will advise you whether this ego trip is worthwhile and, if it is, how to accomplish it safely and effectively.

This chapter won't tell you how to actually write the book. If you plan to write the whole book by yourself (i.e. monograph) then you must generate a certain number of chapters - bound together by a common idea and organized in a logical sequence. If you are to edit a book, your writing task may include 'editorial comments', an 'introduction' and 'conclusion' chapters or a few of the actual chapters. How to write a chapter you have just learned in the previous chapter.

The idea: it has to be original

The idea for your book has to be original. (Originality according to Webster's Third New International Dictionary - is 'the quality of being authentic or genuine, freshness of aspect or design, independence or newness of style or character, novelty in the form of expression'). With the numerous new surgical titles published each year it is almost impossible to be 'original'. But it is a must.

With the latest editions of Schwartz, Sabiston, Greenfield, Baily & Love, Maingot and many other 'classical' textbooks what is your chance of generating another 'original' multi-author text? Probably very low, but not negligible - if you find a gap or generate a new twist. What about yet another comprehensive textbook looking at all the usual topics through the veil of the new gimmick of 'evidence-based surgery'? There won't be a library, or a department, which fails to purchase such a title.

Originality in scientific publishing - as opposed to the non-scientific literary world - is measured in current terms. When what we know may be obsolete in five years your idea has to be original against what is available now - not 10 years ago. For example, looking for an idea for a multi-author text we managed to revive a series on 'Controversies in Surgery'. Such title was available 20 years ago but there was no current competition. Originality may also be expressed in style or tone. A few modern books are available on 'emergency abdominal surgery' but you may choose to do one, say, in verse. We produced such a book using informal, chatty language and much humor. Likewise, there are many texts dedicated to 'surgical infections' - looking at the same topic through the perspective of 'source control' we managed to 'sell' this idea to the publisher as 'original 'and lacking competition.

Examine your book idea against current and past similar titles in the library, bookshop, or on the Internet. Closely scrutinize the competitors. Remember, that you have to be original if you are not an authoritative giant in the field.

The market: who will buy your book?

You need the book for your CV and ego, the publisher needs it in order to survive, but the book is written for the readers and without them, your book is doomed. The rule of thumb is that if your book lacks the potential to sell 1000 copies no publisher will touch it [1]. A surgical title which sells more than 2000 copies is considered a bestseller. Think about yourself - how critical and selective you are when considering buying yet another surgical book. With the numerous titles available, with easily downloadable sources on the Internet, the market for your book is inherently saturated and has to be carefully planned. For example:

◆ If you plan a book which is suitable only to your country (e.g. 'Surgical malpractice in the UK') it has to attract a wide audience: surgeons, surgical trainees, anaesthetists, lawyers and administrators.

◆ If you plan a book on a recent technology (e.g. endovascular stenting) which will be obsolete in a year or two, you have to attract an international surgical and radiological readership. The number of such experts in your country is too small to warrant a book.

◆ On the other hand, a book on basic principles (i.e. 'Common Sense Emergency Abdominal Surgery') may have a longer shelf life but even it may do better if aimed at surgeons and their trainees in an international setting.

◆ The book market is global. Your books may appear in bookshops in Japan, South Africa and India. Do not neglect the international readership. A multi-author book, which neglects British contributors, won't sell well in the UK.

◆ Understand the market limitations when writing in your own language. A German book from Austria could be sold in Germany, Switzerland and 'Germanophile' medical communities elsewhere (e.g. Japan, Turkey). A book in Arabic has a huge potential market. A surgical book in Hebrew, however, will not achieve a significant market.

Can you do it: is the ego trip realistic?

If you were a Professor of Surgery at a major University and a leader in the field, realizing your idea could be relatively easy. Publishers welcome 'big names' who have usually published books before. 'Big names' are well connected and thus can easily procure as many 'top' quality contributors as they wish. They also enjoy an infrastructure including Fellows, research assistants and sectaries. But can the average guy such as yourself do it?

♦ Can you spare the time? Editing or writing a book will take at least a year and usually more than that. Whether you as a full time surgeon can brace yourself for such an arduous task is a question you have to consider before searching for a publisher. Are you willing and able to sacrifice your already scanty leisure time? Not having published a book is not a sin but to abort a book is a sin which may generate ridicule and even enemies.

♦ Will the publisher talk to you? Book publishing is a business and a profession [1]. It is true that publishers prefer 'famous' and established editors/writers but in their constant search for titles they will consider any proposal, including yours. If you plan a monograph then all depends on the novelty and attractiveness of your book proposal. If, on the other hand, you wish to edit a multi-author book the situation is more complex. What makes you qualified to edit a book? Are you an 'authority' in the topic? Will you be able to procure imminent contributors? Will your name 'sell' the book? If the answers to any of these questions are negative, you may want to join force with a more senior and distinguished colleague to serve as your 'active' or 'passive' co-editor. Her or his name may open doors.

The publishers and a book proposal

'They just wanted to sell books...' Bob Dylan wrote and they do. Like your administrators or local HMO's, publishers are there to make money from you. The medical publishers of today are a 'difficult crowd'; having to perform in a world of ever increasing competition, mergers and diminishing revenues. They want you to do all the work for almost nothing in return except having your name on the cover of the book. They want also to dictate the shape and nature of the covers!

Before approaching a publisher you have to have a book proposal. When preparing this bear in mind the principle qualities of an 'ideal book' according to the publishers:

◆ Huge potential market

◆ Current

◆ Durable

Your book proposal has to be brief and neat. Publishers are impatient and they know that if your proposal looks shabby so will your book.

Book Proposal

◆ Title: (e.g. A surgeon's guide to writing and publishing).

◆ A paragraph on what is this book about and why it is 'special' or 'original'?

◆ The market: list all those who may buy it.

◆ The competition: list all similar books available. What makes your book 'better' or 'different'?

◆ Outline: make list of chapters and if a multi-author book provide a provisional list of contributors.

- Format: approximated length of each chapter (pages, words), length of book (pages, words).

- Figures and illustration: number, type, colour?

- About the author/editor: a paragraph about yourself and your previous accomplishments (attach your CV).

Now find a publisher

Unlike submitting an original manuscript for publication you may offer your book proposal simultaneously to many publishers. Do not send your proposal 'blindly' to the publishing house but call or write and ask for the name and address of the commissioning editor responsible for procuring books in your area of interest.

Wait patiently for a reply. It may take a few months during which the commissioning editor checks your credentials, consults with his own surgical 'experts in the field' and together with his product and marketing team, calculates the estimated cost of the project and its profitability.

Do not get discouraged by multiple negative replies. After being rejected by all major medical publishing houses in your country try a smaller publisher or one across the ocean. The publishing market has become global and a small UK publisher, for example, may be able to advertise and sell your book internationally. In general, the smaller the publisher the more personal attention and less arrogance you encounter. Lists of medical publishers are available on the Internet.

Contract & money matters

Once you find a commissioning editor who is genially interested, try to meet her or him face to face; personal chemistry may open a door to many projects in the future. The best opportunities to meet editors are at major international or national surgical meetings. It has been said by Siegfried Unself: 'one of the signs of Napoleon's greatness is the fact that he once had a publisher shot'. But you need your book published so cultivate your editor/publisher and be nice to her or him. Follow, however, John Creasey's advice: 'never buy an editor a lunch or a drink until he has bought a book from you. This is absolute and may be broken at your peril'.

After the lunch or dinner, it is time to talk about the contract. Never ever start the book without a signed contract as in today's world of mergers your publisher of today may not exist next week. A signed contract is not an insurance card for a publisher can decide not to publish a book a year after such a contract was signed.

The contract usually will be a 'standard' one used routinely by the publishers for all scientific books. Most publishers will insist on being provided with an electronic ready for print manuscript and will demand that you are responsible for its accuracy and language. Pay attention, however, to the following details:

- Delivery date: What ever you think add six months.

- Index: This should be generated by the publisher.

- Number of free copies for the Editors and contributors (the contributors will hate you if they are not provided with free copies).

- The shape of the book (hard or paper back) and of the cover.

- Marketing (a painful matter on which you will have little control).

Money? Forget about money! As Jules Renard said: 'writing is the only profession where no one considers you ridiculous if you earn no money'. Unless you are a leading 'giant' in your field the publishers will let you feel that they are doing you a favour. You will spend numerous hours over many years hardly seeing a penny unless your book is a huge bestseller. In the limited realm of surgical publishing this is most unlikely. So you do it for the 'fun and fame!' You might ask for a modest 'advance' for 'administrative expenses'.

Editors vs. Contributors

From the first step the aspiring book editor is wedged between the publishers and the contributing authors. Be nice to your contributors. You may think that you do them a favour by inviting them but in fact it is them who do you a favour by helping with your ego trip for no money and a relatively minor addition to their CV. Remember that for a contributor's CV a book chapter is less valuable than an original paper.

The process of procuring contributors for your book involves a science which has been poorly described hitherto. The ideal contributing author for your multi-authored book is a 'famous giant' in her/his field and an accomplished writer (she has to be, otherwise she would not be 'famous'). Typically however the 'giants' are constantly over committed - a fact, which has the following potential consequences.

- The 'refusnik'. The 'giant' may refuse your invitation. When editing a book, which requires sixty authors, you will get five immediate refusals. Initially your feelings may be hurt - 'what, my book is not important enough for her?' Later you will understand that a polite decline is an honest act which saves you time and frustrations.

- The over committed 'giant' accepts your invitation and immediately delegates the task of writing to his junior colleague. This is fine as long as the 'giant' meaningfully controls the final product. Occasionally it is not so and all you get is a text written by the junior without the touch of novelty and wisdom you expect from the 'giant'. Some 'giants' would commit their name to a sub-optimal chapter they hardly had the time to review.

◆ A few 'giants' may engage in self-plagiarism. This is not uncommon and sadly understandable. Having been invited to write numerous chapters and reviews on their topic of main interest the 'giant' is forced to use his 'mouse' to 'click and paste' whole segments from his previous work onto the new chapter. As long as the new chapter is good this is not a disaster as 'patchy' self-plagiarism of purely educational material is not considered an ethical misconduct.

◆ The 'fugitive' giant. Even 'giants' may first accept the invitation to contribute and then totally ignore all your efforts to procure the chapter from them. Your 'reminder' letters, e-mails and even phone calls are never returned and you will never see their chapter. You start wondering how they ever became 'giants'. The incidence of such disasters is fortunately rare (around 5% per book) but when it occurs it is time consuming and may significantly delay the submission of the book to print.

◆ 'Giants' are often late. Characteristically, they start writing the chapter only after the deadline arrives.

Most 'giants', however, will provide on schedule an excellent, well-written and well-polished chapter.

An alternative to the 'giants' are 'upcoming talents'. These are younger but talented academicians who strive to establish their names. You can identify them in a MEDLINE search, during society meetings, in journals and in major textbooks - where their names may be overshadowed by their 'giant-mentor' co-authors.

Practical tips for the inexperienced editor

◆ Strive for a balanced combination of 'giants' and 'upcoming talents'; give a chance to relatively unknown surgeons because they may surprise you with the quality of their product. In order to satisfy your publisher at least half of the contributors have to be 'giants'.

◆ Maintain a list of 'excellent contributors' and use them repeatedly. This is, however, impossible when your books focus on an ever-changing set of topics. Similarly, have a black list of those who are habitually late and/or poor writers. Try not to use them again. Never re-invite a 'fugitive' contributor. On the other hand, you may invite a 'refusnik' again because your new invitation may be of a greater interest.

◆ Always get yourself a few 'spare' chapters for every book and you will not have to worry about 'no shows' any more.

◆ Always overestimate the time required to produce a book. You will never have all the chapters on your desk earlier than six months after the declared deadline. The more 'complex' is your project, the longer it will take to print, the more outdated your book will be when it appears.

◆ Be careful when inviting authors from non-English speaking countries. Be sure that they know how to write English or be ready to translate their work from Italian - English or American English to 'true' English-English. US and UK based readers and reviewers are very sensitive and critical.

◆ Provide the contributors with a well-structured outline of the book, specific requirements for the individual chapters and a sample chapter written by you. Assume, however, that most contributors will not follow your instructions. They will need repeated reminders.

Be obsessive with your editorial process. The responsibility for the final product is fully yours.

The anti-climax

Alfred Kazin wrote: '... the publishing of his ideas, though it brings gratifications, is a curious anticlimax'. Remember that transient void one feels after a nine-hour operation or an excellent meal. The same can happen after your book eventually appears. As Tim Albert writes: 'Your mother will be proud, you will get the odd review, most of which these days tend to be full of faint praise. Your colleagues are unlikely to be too enthusiastic....' [2].

But who cares about jealous colleagues or money when you can smell and hug your fresh book. A few words from a young surgeon such as 'I read your excellent book' will compensate you for the long hours. Your book may even become a classic - calling for additional editions.

'For several days after my first book was published I carried it around in my pocket and took a surreptitious peek at it to make sure the ink had not faded'.
Sir James M. Barrie

References

1   Banks M. Get your book published. *BMJ* 1998; 317: 1715-1718.
2   Albert T. How to become a book author. *BMJ* 2000; 320: S2-7237.

Commentary
by L. M. Nyhus
Warren H. Cole Professor and Head of the Department of Surgery, Emeritus, University of Illinois College of Medicine, Chicago, U.S.A.

My deadline for preparing this 'Comment' is fast approaching. Since the tardy conributor is well-defined in the chapter, I do not wish to be placed in the category of the 'often late' participant and move forward toward an on-time submission.

Having edited over 95 surgical texts including new editions and foreign translations (Spanish, German, Portugese, Polish, Japanese, French) I can vouch for the many points of wisdom succinctly presented in this chapter.

The beginning
Near the completion of my surgical residency, my chief Professor Henry N. Harkins of the University of Washington, Seattle suggested that I spend a year of study overseas at centres known for work in the field of gastrointestinal physiology and surgery. We had written numerous scientific papers in this area and it was Dr. Harkins' belief that from additional material collected overseas we might edit a book.

I studied with Professor Philip Sandblom in Lund, Sweden and Professor Sir Charles Illingworth in Glasgow,

Scotland. The scene was set and we published 'Surgery of the Stomach and Duodenum' in 1962.

This text was successful and is currently in its 5th edition with a modified title, 'Surgery of the Esophagus, Stomach and Small Intestine'. It is obvious that I stumbled upon a truism as presented by Schein. I began this long editorial journey by joining 'giant' Harkins who taught me much of what is in the Schein text. As an aside, having produced a successful first edition of a given book, subsequent editions were much easier to collate than the first. Unfortunately, most books find no brothers or sisters on the library shelf following a one and only edition.

Additional observations

'Giants are often late'. I would be remiss if I did bow to my 'giant' authors. Robert M. Zollinger, Sr., of Ohio State University was prominent in many of my books. Was he a busy person? Of course, but he was always the first to submit his chapter well ahead of the deadline. The list of those 'greats' who are attentive to publishing deadlines is long: we youngsters should note.

Contract and money matters

The major textbooks of surgery can earn significant monetary return. Several surgery texts have circulations of over 100,000 copies per edition. Most specialty books are successful (from the publisher point of view) if sales reach 2500 copies. The standard royalty to editors is 10 percent on up to 7500-10,000 copies and most publishing houses will increase the royalty to 12.5 percent for the next 2500-5000 copies sold. This possible escalation of royalty distribution should be discussed at contract development time. The distribution of royalty cheques is a happy occasion in the life of a successful editor.

Copyright date

Don't allow the publisher to complete your book for sale in a late month of a given year without giving the next year as the date of publication. Medical books age rapidly and a three year old book may be considered out-of-date. A surgical book shown for the first time at the American College of Surgeons Congress in October may have a copyright date in the following year. This may be a small point, but it recognizes the need to prevent unfair early ageing of a book's life. Only by forethought can an astute editor assure manuscript flow for timely presentation of the finished product at the Congress of Surgeons.

The anti-climax

I do not understand this concept. My excitement and pride escalated upon receipt of each new book. From the raw material presented to the publisher, the final product was always improved and a joy to behold.

The ultimate climax for editors might be the award of a prize. Robert J. Baker and I received the H. H. Hawkins Award in 1984 for the first edition of 'Mastery of Surgery'. This award is the Grand Prize given annually by the Professional and Scholarly Division of the Association of American Publishers for the Outstanding Technical, Scientific or Medical Book of the year. There is no chance for anti-climax here.

Chapter
14

Chapter 15

How to write a commentary

A. Fingerhut

Chief of Service, Digestive Surgery

Centre Hospitalier Intercommunal, Poissy, France

&

Associate Professor of Surgery

Louisiana State University Medical School

New Orleans, LA, U.S.A.

This job usually falls to an expert in the field and/or a 'big name'. You may be invited to write a commentary arising from the fact that you recently wrote a paper or gave a lecture on the same topic. It is similar in structure to an 'editorial' or a 'letter to the editor'. However, being asked to write a commentary means one of two things and places you in one of two categories:

◆ either the authors/editors of a book want your name somewhere but forgot to ask you to write a chapter or could not get you on the author's list for other reasons, or

◆ your sense of analysis and critique is such that the organizer of a meeting or the editors of a book prefer to have your commentary because they think it is as valuable as a chapter contribution.

In the first instance, do not be offended, this is the perfect occasion to make a brilliant intervention and quickly rise to become a full-fledged member of the second category!

You may be asked to write a commentary in two different settings. One is the 'written' version of an oral commentary made at the end of an oral presentation delivered in surgical meetings such as the American Surgical Association or the European Surgical Association. This is sometimes also called an 'invited commentary'. The author is often called the 'discussant', a term I shall use indifferently for either type of presentation. The oral part of the communication is best prepared as a previously written text and this should correspond exactly to what is said orally. Because the 'oral' commentary subsequently goes to press this means that the message will be permanent. The other is a commentary to a chapter of a book, much like what you may find at the end of one of the chapters in this work.

The commentary is divided into three (and sometimes four) parts:

◆ state the goals the authors set for themselves and how they went about their work (patients and methods);

◆ indicate whether they have attained the goals and why;

- add your personal experience on the matter and/or a brief review of the literature and comment how the authors' results fit into this framework.

- In the version corresponding to an invited commentary of an oral presentation there may be one or several questions.

Preparing your commentary means that you should dispose of at least the summary, but ideally the text, well in advance in order to be able to make pertinent remarks and comments. When accepting the invitation, even if the summary is sent quickly, you should ask for the full text to be forwarded as soon as possible. Beware of short delays, the time necessary to write a good commentary may compromise your already busy schedule. Do not hesitate to contact the author directly.

Thanking the authors for the opportunity of commenting on their presentation or text is unnecessary but may sometimes be politically correct (essentially in the invited commentary form). Thanks often go to the authors who were kind enough to send their text to you well in advance. While often seen in the commentary at the end of an article in a journal, this is hardly ever necessary in the written form at the end of a book chapter.

Stating the goals of the authors is usually straightforward.

Next comes the brief statement of how the authors proceeded to achieve their goals and discuss their results and/or conclusions. Only the essential points should be highlighted: there is no place for too many details.

The essence of the commentary is emphasizing the strong points of the study or work and arguing how it agrees or disagrees with common thought, literature, the discussant's experience or any combination thereof. It may well be the occasion to add something that the authors may have missed or ignored, that you feel is important. Do not use this invitation, however, to cite your own personal list of references. One or two references to your own publications or research on the topic is usually enough to make your point. You, as an expert in the field, usually have already dealt with the topic; this is probably why you were chosen to do the job of commenting, and there should be no further need to 'show off' in this manner.

Here your job is to detail one or more of the strong points, state whether they are credible, whether they are in keeping with the methods employed to attain them, and whether they concur with the literature. If you agree with any or all of these points, then be brief; if you disagree then you have to elaborate on why this is so.

Remember that the quality of the commentary is in the pertinence of the remarks and is inversely proportional to its length.

You must not lose sight of your role and you must not take the place of the speaker or writer. A commentary differs from an editorial in that the text here must be complementary to the original text. It differs from the letter to the editor in which the author of the letter nearly always has something critical to say. In the oral version of an invited commentary, the functions of the discussant are to emphasize and highlight the qualities of the communication and to stimulate the beginning of the discussion in the meeting. In both types of commentaries, the goals are to highlight the strong points (whether they originate from the original report or from the commentary) and bring them into perspective with the message meant by the original authors.

There should be no more than three or four pertinent references. Try not to use the same as those already cited in the original paper.

The presentation given orally may differ slightly from the text you have received because there is often a time span between the deadline for the authors' text and the actual date of the presentation. The text to be published is written and/or corrected after the presentation has taken place. Therefore, ask for the final version of the text before submitting your final comments to make sure that everything corresponds, and that eventual changes in the text have not altered the meaning of your commentary.

Chapter 16

On the editor's desk

J. R. Farndon

Professor and Head of Division, University of Bristol
& Consultant Surgeon, Bristol Royal Infirmary, Bristol, UK.

J. A. Murie

Consultant Vascular Surgeon & Honorary Senior Lecturer
Royal Infirmary of Edinburgh, Edinburgh, UK

This chapter describes 'the moment of decision'.

So far this book has brought you from the reasons to write and from the first germ of an idea, through the difficulties and tribulations of writing, to the business of sending the final product for editorial assessment. The first section of this chapter deals with issues specific to the *British Journal of Surgery* and the second considers more general editorial matters.

An obvious place to begin is to ask: 'Who and what are editors?' In the case of the *BJS* the editors are chosen and appointed by the British Journal of Surgery Society, a charity that is formally registered as a limited company, with audited accounts and statutory business meetings. No doubt preceding editors advise on suitable successors; the two current editors have worked up the ladder from referee, through associate editor, to their current position. The editors are not themselves members of the Council of the British Journal of Surgery Society; if this were the case they would be in the awkward position of overseeing their own terms and conditions of service. It is observed that editors of other surgical journals frequently emerge from editorial boards.

The overall direction and strategy of the Journal comes from the Editorial Committee almost as a mission statement: 'The *British Journal of Surgery* features the very best in clinical and laboratory-based research on all aspects of general surgery and related topics. Developing areas such as minimally invasive therapy and interventional radiology are strongly represented.' (See 'Aims and Scope', in the Journal Frontispiece). The editors are also involved in developments and innovations, such as new article formats and electronic mechanisms (web site and article submission, referencing and publication, etc). The bulk of an editor's work, however, is the day to day management of articles and letters received for consideration for publication.

The *BJS* editor's desk

Your article or letter will be read by at least one editor upon receipt and the immediate division is that reviews, leaders and vascular articles are dealt with by John Murie and the rest by John Farndon (editors). Articles may be sent to any of the associate editors (Jonothan Earnshaw, Pierre Guillou and Ronan O'Connell) for a specialist opinion or to Gordon Murray for statistical advice. They are then sent out to two or (usually) three referees. The number of articles rejected immediately at editorial level is about 5% and comprises case reports (note: we do not seek these in our current state of excellent copy flow of high quality articles) and articles that are inappropriate for the readership of the Journal (e.g. a new method of internal fixation of fractures of the fibula). Articles for immediate rejection are nearly always cross-checked between editors. No unsolicited article is accepted on editorial opinion alone.

If your article is one of the 95% of papers that we receive (1200-1400 per year), read and send out to referees, we acknowledge receipt of your manuscript and choose referees to evaluate your work. This choice must be made carefully and objectively, and depends largely on the main theme of the article. Other clues that may help select suitable referees can be obtained from the bibliography, but care is needed to avoid sending an article submitted by Smidgin to be refereed by Buggins, when the article from Smidgin has discredited Buggins' life's work. The editors read almost 4000 reports each year from a panel of 1000 supportive *BJS* referees. We know who are hawks and who are doves. We know the degrees of concordance between our referees [1], and know that there is little difference between whether you or we choose the referees to the eventual outcome of the decision making process [2]. Referees provide a main report in free text plus a confidential report that relies greatly on objective scoring (Fig 1). We place great store in this attempt at objectivity. A paper may obtain straight 'A's in importance of topic, analysis, presentation, etc., but it will be rejected if it has an 'E' for novelty. The decision to accept or reject is usually easy and based on referee opinion; hanging judges are only rarely required from the Editorial Committee to reconcile widely differing reports. Difficult files are always discussed at the monthly meeting of the editors.

FIGURE 1
The British Journal of Surgery
Referee's Report Form

The British Journal of Surgery
Referee's Report Form
Confidential Comments for the Editors

These are comments made in strict confidence to the *British Journal of Surgery* and will not be transmitted directly to the author(s), but may be used to aid revision of the manuscript.

This form is available for electronic submission from the *BJS* website (www.bjs.co.uk).

Reviewer's Details
Name:
Email:
Date:
Manuscript Details
Number:
Title:
Author(s):

Assessment

Please grade each feature (where appropriate) from A (excellent) to E (very poor):

	A	B	C	D	E
Novelty/originality	☐	☐	☐	☐	☐
Clinical importance	☐	☐	☐	☐	☐
Scientific importance	☐	☐	☐	☐	☐
Analysis of data	☐	☐	☐	☐	☐
Presentation/grammar/style	☐	☐	☐	☐	☐

(including illustrations, tables, etc.)

Abstract

Does the summary give an adequate picture   Yes ☐   No ☐

of the paper overall?

Introduction

Are the aims and objectives of the paper   Yes ☐   No ☐

set out *succinctly*?

Are the aims and objectives of the paper   Yes ☐   No ☐

set out *clearly*?

Materials and methods

Are these clearly explained?   Yes ☐   No ☐

Are the methods easily understood?   Yes ☐   No ☐

Results

Are adequate numbers used?   Yes ☐   No ☐

Is the statistical method appropriate?   Yes ☐   No ☐

Are statistics necessary?   Yes ☐   No ☐

Discussion and conclusions

Are the conclusions clearly stated?   Yes ☐   No ☐

Are the conclusions justified?   Yes ☐   No ☐

Are there any ethical issues to be addressed?   Yes ☐   No ☐

Are the conclusions adequately discussed   Yes ☐   No ☐

against the background of current and health issues?

Recommendation

Please give an overall score to the paper where:

☐   A - excellent, must publish

☐   B - good but needs minor correction

☐   C - correctable deficits, probably publish

☐   D - major faults? reject

☐   E - very poor, reject outright

Additional Comments for the Editor

Please use this space to write any confidential comments to the Editor

If a paper obtains marginal support, the editor will examine the manuscript once more, assess whether the criticisms are correctable, and will tend to err on the side of encouragement. Most articles are returned for corrections and for authors to attend to referees' comments. Sometimes a hint of gloom will pervade the accompanying letter, 'You will see that our referees felt your article was seriously flawed.', or a glimmer of hope will be provided, 'If you do resubmit your article ... etc'.

Errors of judgement in either direction occur infrequently. An article can end up on an associate editor's desk being prepared for publication after an editor and three referees have all failed to spot glaring errors. This usually occurs when the theme of an article is in the associate editor's specialty area. The initial decision to accept has to be reversed and the paper will be rejected with regrets and apologies. The Journal receives a challenge to its decision in less than 1% of rejected articles. If the arguments presented by the authors requesting re-examination are cogent and objective, the paper may be reviewed again and usually by different referees who are not party to the past history of the paper.

The current acceptance rate of about 20% reflects standards provided mainly by the referees. The editors have not adjusted the set point of acceptance/rejection in the last 5 years. With this strategy, and by concentrating on more substantial scientific papers, the citation index and impact factor of the Journal are rising. Once accepted, the editors work with authors to polish the manuscript before typesetting. You may be asked to resubmit attending further to points raised by referees and one or more editors. The resubmission will be checked again by an editor to ensure that referees' criticisms have been met and a final buff to high shine will be made to unify English, grammar, style and layout.

The editors hope that significant learning accrues even from rejected articles. Referees' comments are usually fed back to authors and these may help to re-craft the paper prior to submission to another journal. Hopefully, if the criticisms are profound the authors realise the need to do more work rather than attempt immediate resubmission. Although two or three referees' reports may be received, these are not all sent out to authors - a minority are of little use and some are too terse! Referees see reports from fellow referees specific for each article to provide bench marking and hopefully to drive up the quality of the referee process.

The editor's desk cannot be tidy and effective without an efficient support team, and those in John Street are just such. We also meet regularly with our publisher, Blackwell Science, at away days in Oxford, exploring new methods and techniques to be implemented in editing and producing a journal of this century (see below).

The editor's desk in general

Editors want to receive high quality papers that need minimal hands-on attention. Editors everywhere are aware of the fragility of the peer review process and that:

'1   'Chiding' reviews to authors do not usefully improve quality.

2   Exchanging reviews has no effect on quality of review.

3   Reviewers aged 40 or less and those trained in epidemiology and statistics write better reviews.

4   Bias and parochialism can be found in most peer review systems and

5   Developing an instrument to measure manuscript quality remains the greatest challenge.' [3]

Internet peer review is an emerging editorial function that is acceptable to most authors and reviewers but this does not provide an adequate substitute for the commissioned pre-publication review. Points in favour of pre-publication internet review are that editors receive input from wide and unexpected sources and the internet system allows readers to gain some insight into the whole process [4].

Editors must ensure that only work of high quality, with carefully described and tested methodology, is published. An article with poor methodology may produce skewed or erroneous end results and recommendations. Clinical practice may be affected by such a publication with serious consequences, or significant effects may be produced in a meta-analysis [5].

Occasionally major pieces of work that have already been published are discredited. A recent example concerned a study of high-dose chemotherapy in patients with high risk primary breast cancer (Bezwoda and associates). Peer review and the editorial process was not an essential component of the conduct of the clinical work [6] and editors must be forgiven for not spotting this type of fraud. This could only have been prevented if there was international registration of clinical trials with continuous monitoring of quality assurance [7]. In an attempt to improve the quality of research some journals provide prospective advice on the structure and content of the proposed work before it begins, but without a definite commitment to publish any subsequent papers which may emanate from the work. Editors have a duty to declare openly any publishing misdemeanour detected within their domain and the *BJS* has been pre-eminent in this activity. Professor Farthing writes later in this book on the ethics of publication.

Editors must look forward and be ready to embrace new technology. Most journals already ask for manuscripts to be submitted on disk and many (including *BJS*) are able to offer on-line submission. The latter has obvious convenience in terms of reducing the size of postal packets between author and editor; it has not yet, however, obviated the need for standard mail altogether (signed letters of submission and certain illustrations still need to be sent by the old method). The 'electronic manuscript' is also convenient within a journal office. It can be sent on-line to any editor for choice of referees and, at a later stage, for decision making in terms of acceptance or rejection. Increasingly, editors are actually editing on-line and the internal office use of paper is diminishing; at least that is the goal.

In the future, will it be essential to have your work on four glossy pages of *BJS* before anyone even begins to think about its credibility? Open internet peer review on the road to publication is one thing, but is the clinical scientific community ready for the e-print - a preliminary publication posted on a website that anyone can read and digest? E-print servers exist in some specialty areas, such as astronomy, and the *British Medical Journal* has recently posed the question: if you put up an article on a website would this be publication? [8] Would you want the work endorsed later by paper publication? The *BMJ* has stated that the prior posting as an e-print would not preclude definitive paper publication: 'this is the age of transparency rather than paternalism' (Richard Smith, *BMJ* editor). The concept is developed further by Tony Delamothe (*BMJ* web editor) and Richard Smith [9] who describe how 'their' journal, in partnership with Stanford University Libraries, will establish an e-print server. It is hoped that this will invigorate the review process, producing a higher quality end product which could still be paper published. 'The e-print looks like the first substantially new form of scientific communication since the peer reviewed article, and as we're in the business of transmitting scientific information, it makes sense for us to work to find the e-print's right place in the new digital environment. ... We may find that we lose our jobs or have to accept reduced salaries if the BMJ Publishing Group becomes unprofitable because of proposals like that from the National Institutes of Health [9].'

References

1   Farndon JR, Murie JA, Johnson CD, Earnshaw JJ, Guillou PJ. The referee process of the British Journal of Surgery - Editorial. *Br J Surg* 1997; 84: 901-903.

2   Earnshaw JJ, Farndon JR, Guillou PJ, Johnson CD, Murie JA, Murray GD. A comparison of reports from referees chosen by authors or journal editors in the peer review process. *Ann R Coll Surg Engl* 2000 Apr; 82 (4 Suppl): 133-135.

3   Goldbeck-Wood S. Evidence on peer review - scientific quality control or smokescreen? *Br Med J* 1999; 318: 44-45.

4   Bingham CM, Higgins G, Coleman R, Van Der Weyden MB. The Medical Journal of Australia internet peer-review study. *The Lancet* 1998; 352: 441-445.

5   Moher D, et al. Does quality of reports of randomised trials affect estimates of intervention efficacy reported in meta-analyses? *The Lancet* 1998; 352: 609-613.

6   Weiss RB, et al. High-dose chemotherapy for high-risk primary breast cancer: an on-site review of the Bezwoda study. *The Lancet* 2000; 355: 999-1003.

7   Horton R. Commentary - After Bezwoda. *The Lancet* 2000; 355: 942-943.

8   Smith R. Editorial - What is publication? *Br Med J* 1999; 318: 142.

9   Delamothe T, Smith R. Moving beyond journals: the future arrives with a crash. *Br Med J* 1999; 318: 1637-1639.

Commentary
by A. E. Baue

Professor Emeritus of Surgery, Vice President for the Medical Center, Emeritus, Saint Louis University School of Medicine, St. Louis, Missouri, U.S.A.

Drs. Farndon and Murie provide an excellent account of the work and responsibilities of editors of a surgical journal and how journals function. Their chapter is an example of what the late A. Bartlett Giamatti said - ' . . .

expressing the results of that thinking, in speech and in writing, with clarity, logic, and grace.'[1] An editor has a great responsibility to the readers and writers who have trusted their manuscripts to the journal. Someone worked hard to produce the manuscript and they should be encouraged. As an editor, I also felt more humble than powerful. I was reminded of T. S. Eliot saying, 'Some editors are failed writers but so are most writers'[2] or the observation of Adlai Stevenson that 'An editor is one who separates the wheat from the chaff and publishes the chaff.'[3] It is easier to publish chaff because wheat is often controversial. I agree that the fate of a manuscript may be determined by the choice of referees. Editors must know referees: some accept everything, some reject everything ('hawks and doves,'[3] as described), but most are balanced and thoughtful in their reviews. I never used the word reject in writing to authors but rather 'Your manuscript has not been accepted for publication . . . .' and gave reasons and comments of the reviewers.[4] Reviewers' comments were edited if they were sarcastic or critical of the authors rather than the manuscript. Should reviewers remain anonymous? I think so. Otherwise, they may not be critical. I published several manuscripts rejected by prominent editorial board members because they did not fit in with their perceptions.[5] I asked them to write editorial comments with the manuscripts which they did with subdued comments. Farndon and Murie refer to Smidgin and Buggins. There are suggestions for writers and reviewers by Farndon and Murie which I emphasize:

the title is the message not the medium; is an incomplete bibliography poor scholarship or sour grapes?; research papers take a bigger beating in the review process than do clinical reports; being a reviewer is a labor of love for surgery; have something worthwhile to say (do not report the 15th case of Tsu Tsu Gamushi's disease in the Antarctic unless you have important or new observations); detailed comments for authors help them; writing a good abstract is not abstract writing; the most important part of writing is rewriting.[6]

The quotation, 'Your manuscript is both good and original. Unfortunately, what is original is not good and what is good is not original' is attributed to Samuel Johnson.

Bibliography

1   Giamatti AB. The earthly use of a liberal education. *Yale Alumni Magazine* 1983; 67: 42-44.

2   Eliot TS cited by M Stephens. In: M Stephens (ed). *Dictionary of Literary Quotations*. New York, NY: Rutledge, 1990.

3   Stephenson A. Ibid. 95.

4   Baue AE. Reflections of a former editor. *Arch Surg* 1993; 128: 1305-1314.

5   Baue AE. Peer and/or Peerless Review. *Arch Surg* 1985; 120: 880-888.

6   Baue AE. Writing an abstract is not abstract writing. *Arch Surg* 1979; 114: 11-12.

Chapter 17

Politics
in surgical
publishing

C. J. Laitman

Senior Editor and Managing Editor, Annals of Surgery
University of Wisconsin Medical School
Clinical Science Center, Madison, Wisconsin, U.S.A.

L. F. Rikkers

A.R. Curreri Professor and Chairman
Department of Surgery
University of Wisconsin Medical School
Clinical Science Center, Madison, Wisconsin, U.S.A.

So far, this book has dealt with factors involving primarily the surgeon-cum-writer. These are the *abcs*, so to speak, of getting started: 'why' to publish an academic surgery paper, and 'what' and 'where' and 'how'. Despite the fact that these aspects of publication create the substance and 'guts' of any paper, they are not the only determinants of the success or failure of a publication effort.

Beyond the individual surgeon-author's efforts or control is the real-world consideration of virtually every social interaction - politics. Politics has been variously defined as 'the art and science of government' and 'intrigue and manoeuvring within a group'. Politics affects academic publishing when individuals, in one way or another, attempt to exert influence on policy or outcome based on personal interests or biases. Politicking, as such, can be manifest from the author's side of the publishing interaction or from the journal's.

Politics in the author's camp

Authorship

The politics of publishing is perhaps nowhere more obvious than in the assignment of authorship. While the person who conceives an idea, gets the funding and does the most work is indisputably entitled to first authorship, other individuals who are granted coauthorship by no means always contribute equitably.

In a nod to patriarchy, the senior faculty member or division/department Chair is frequently made a coauthor on studies to which he or she has made no discernible contribution. This may be academic homage, but it is not honest. The name of a senior faculty member who has contributed to a study is customarily listed last in the order of authors. Other individuals contributing to the study are generally listed after the first author, in descending order of the contribution made.

Others may be awarded coauthorship as a personal thank you, such as individuals representing commercial sponsors for research. The bottom line is that authorship should never be 'for sale'. It must be reserved only for those who make an active and substantial contribution to the study being reported.

This prescript extends to the unsavoury practice of including as authors individuals whose professional renown will add credibility to the work but who have no knowledge of the work or of the use to which their names are being put. People who do this may believe it is a win-win situation, with the unwitting author having another publication to his or her name. In fact, it constitutes fraudulent use of someone else's reputation and, in fact, the person whose name has been used might well find substantial fault with the work being proffered.

Duplicate publication and 'salami-slicing'

Salami-slicing is the practice of cutting up a body of data to yield several papers where one complete paper would be optimal. It may also be used to give several participants in a study a chance at first authorship, often in different specialty journals. Duplicate publication, submitting the same (or substantially the same) study to more than one journal, is done for the same reason. In a system based on quantity rather than quality of papers published, researchers boost their 'counts' by spreading the word as far as it will go.

While the dishonesty inherent to falsifying data is obvious, many people wink at duplicate publication and even more so at 'salami-slicing'. Although acknowledging that these practices are unethical, George Lundberg, former editor of *The Journal of the American Medical Association*, described the differences as follows. If falsifying data is 'a felony with intent to commit vehicular homicide, then duplicate publication would be a traffic ticket' [1]. Nevertheless, such 'misdemeanours' are not without price.

Although all reputable journals have policies against these practices, their prevalence is all too widespread - up to 25 per cent of the published literature by some estimates [2]. So what's the harm? For one, it is an ongoing problem for editors who are constantly wrestling with publisher-imposed page limitations, and with the professional and ethical responsibility to optimize the use of available pages. Scientifically, redundant publication is detrimental since it tends to overestimate the effects of whatever drugs, techniques or interventions are being discussed. Such distortions may lead to misuse of the proposed treatments, or misallocation of research and clinical resources. This short-changes everyone.

Politics in the journal's camp

Peer review process

At its best, 'peer review weeds out bad studies and recognizes good ones' [3] but the process is far from perfect.

Reviewers may be biased. For example, they might downgrade a manuscript sent to them for review if the content of the paper contravenes what they themselves practise. Or they may be biased in favour of (or against) a particular institution or researcher. One study showed that editors and reviewers favoured prestigious authors, and made more allowances for male authors [4]. A solution would be to double-blind the review process or to open it up completely. This issue is not likely to be resolved in the immediate future.

Reviewers may lack the expertise to evaluate a paper sent to them. Science has become so specialized that even professionals in the same field may well not be knowledgeable about a subspecialty area. Yet it is the perversity of human nature - and surgeons are surely not immune - that we are loath to admit ignorance, especially in situations in which professional egos may be on the line. To those reviewers who are notable exceptions and let us know that they are out of their professional depth for reviewing a particular manuscript, we tip our hats and extend our admiration.

Reviewers may be too busy to provide a careful review. Many of the best known academic surgeons are asked to serve on many editorial boards and they seldom decline. The process would be better served by including more, perhaps less well known but highly capable, surgeons. Those asked to review papers for top surgery journals are generally the most professionally active, frequently with 70-hour working weeks and still not enough time to accomplish everything. A request from a journal editor to review a manuscript or to serve on the editorial board, although flattering, is one more responsibility on already overflowing plates. A recent study showed that review quality increased with increasing time spent on the review, up to but not more than 3 hours [5].

It is the editor's responsibility to resolve any questions of review quality, thoroughness or fairness, usually by obtaining additional reviews.

Commercial sponsorship of submitted works

Financial pressures to order the medical agenda also exist in the form of for-profit sponsorship of medical research. It is an irony of drug regulation that the burden of proof of safety and effectiveness rests with the very companies (pharmaceutical or medical device) that stand to profit most. Perhaps because of this, pharmaceutical companies and manufacturers of medical devices offer financial support to academic scientists for expert evaluation of new products. But such academic partnerships also lend prestige and credibility to the commercial sponsor, warranted or not.

The political challenges are clear. On the one hand, the researcher who accepts support money from a commercial sponsor must take scrupulous care to remain scientifically objective and not succumb to the temptation to identify with the benefactor. The researcher must also resist the temptation to reward financial support with authorship. When the results of a commercially sponsored study are submitted for consideration to a peer-reviewed journal, it must be identified as such. On the other side of the publishing equation, the journal editor must take great care that the sponsorship of any study is clearly stated on the first printed page so that readers can take that into account when deciding on the work's validity. The editor also has the obligation to question authorships if any doubt exists as to propriety.

The editor

Editors and referees, it has been said, are the 'gate-keepers' of science [6]. They have also been variously accused of ignorance, carelessness and even deliberate obstructiveness; of conceptual inbreeding; and gaining an unfair research advantage by having advance access to new research. The truth is more mundane, being somewhere between the exalted and the damned. Editors do help set the medical agenda; it is intrinsic to the job.

Editors choose who will review a paper and, as Arthur Baue pointed out [7], 'the fate of a manuscript can be determined by the selection of reviewers'. A conscientious editor will be aware of the shortcomings as well as the strengths of potential reviewers and will try to achieve a balance. Although the decision to accept or reject a manuscript is often clear, there are many borderline cases and the editor holds ultimate sway over what gets published and what does not.

When, in spite of our best attempts to be fair, an author of a rejected manuscript requests (or sometimes demands) reconsideration, we need to be very honest with ourselves and decide whether there is a legitimate gripe, and proceed accordingly. Not often, but at least on several occasions, truly excellent manuscripts have emerged from this sequence of rejection-reconsideration-acceptance.

The editor's agenda-setting function also extends to who is invited to be a member of the editorial board. This can influence not only what individual papers get published, but what scientific interests and subspecialties are emphasized.

Finally, perhaps the most politically blatant scenario of the editorial office occurs when a prominent academician attempts to influence an editorial decision to accept, or to advance the priority of, a paper in assignment for publication.

Conclusion

It has been suggested that the social context of science operates to control the communication of science [8]. This is but another way of saying that politicking is as inevitable in scientific publishing as it is in any human enterprise. What we must remember, whether as authors or as editors, is that temptations will always exist to advance our more self-serving aims, whether they be small or large. What we must strive for, consciously and consistently, is intellectual honour. The greater good hangs in the balance.

References

1   Lundberg G. Ethics in medical editing. Presentation at the University of Wisconsin-Madison. 29 March, 1999.

2   Jefferson T. Redundant publication in biomedical sciences: scientific misconduct or necessity? *Science and Engineering Ethics* 1998; 4: 135-40.

3   Angell M. Q and A on peer review. *Association of American Medical Colleges Reports.* April 1999; 8: 3.

4   Petty RE & Fleming MA. The review process at PSPB; correlates of inter-reviewer agreement and manuscript acceptance. *Personality and Social Psychology Bulletin* 1999; 25: 188-203.

5   Black N, van Rooyen S, Godlee F, Smith R & Evans S. What makes a good reviewer and a good review for a general medical journal? *JAMA* 1998; 280: 231-3.

6   Campanario JM. On influential books and journal articles initially rejected because of negative referees' evaluations. *Science Communication* 1995; 16: 304-25.

7   Baue A. Refections of a former editor. *Arch Surg.* 1993; 128: 1305-14.

8   Fuller S. The social psychology of scientific knowledge. In: Shadish, WR & Fuller S, eds. *The Social Psychology of Science.* New York: Guilford Press, 1994: 162-78.

Commentary
by M. W. Büchler

Professor of Surgery, Chairman, Department of General Surgery, University of Heidelberg, Heidelberg, Germany

Authorship: patriarchy versus responsible control

Patriarchy in authorship assignment may be a problem in surgical departments with a major research interest in which young surgeons struggle for papers to fulfil academic career requirements. Control and responsibility over primary and secondary data to be submitted for publication from clinical trials or the research laboratory must be maintained. The final control must rest with the senior author. This is particularly the case when dealing with retrospective/prospective material. There may be a tendency to polish (not falsify) without intention. This control is preventive and corrective at the same time. The junior writer should acknowledge this function of the senior author. This control function must occur in the supervising of the resubmission process. In the interest of honesty the balance between positive patriarchy and assignment of senior (corresponding) authorship must be obtained to encourage the development of junior researchers.

Journal ranking and impact factor

In the Journal Citation Reports of 1999 for 'surgery' 130 journals are listed. Within the 15 highest ranked journals 13 are American based and 2 non-American based. Is this difference to be explained by quality issues or is this in part an issue of politics in surgical publishing?

Journal ranking is based on citation and impact factor. American surgical journals receive more citations than others partly because of quality issues but in addition there are some other possible explanations.

1) The leading (impact factor) surgical journal, the Annals of Surgery, publishes a considerable portion of its monthly editions as meeting proceedings of major surgical societies. The leading European surgical journal (Br J Surg) works almost exclusively on submitted and peer reviewed articles. This policy of publishing papers from meetings certainly influences citations because these papers are often the newest and most attractive contributions in surgical science and, if they go into print rapidly, this guarantees citations.

2) Academic surgical careers are frequently determined by qualified publications in the surgical literature. The criterion for such quality is often journal ranking and some universities, for example, only rank papers in the best 10% of the journal category (i.e. the first 13 of 130 surgical journals in ISI ranking). Surgeons, therefore, attempt to publish their papers in such journals for career reasons.

3) Citation as a quality factor results from publishing good papers but is also influenced by marketing and monopoly markets as political instruments.

Conclusion

Laitman and Rikkers are correct in that 'what we must strive for is intellectual honour' and that 'the greater good hangs in the balance'.

References

1   Laitman CJ, Rikkers LF. Politics in Surgical Publishing. *Br J Surg.* 2000; 87: 1284-1286.

Chapter 18

Dealing with the rejected article

P. J. Guillou

Dean of the School of Medicine, University of Leeds

&

Professor of Surgery

St. James's University Hospital, Leeds, UK

J. J. Earnshaw

Consultant Surgeon, Gloucestershire Royal Hospital

Gloucester, UK

Unfortunately the rejection of a submitted article happens to us all at some time or another. Indeed it is fair to say that journal editors initially reject the vast majority of scientific publications and it is the author's response to the comments of editors and referees that determines whether or not an article is ultimately published. Because very few 'first submissions' are published without further modification, the rejection of a manuscript should not be regarded as a personal criticism directed at the author by the referees and editors.

Read the rejection letter carefully

How then to proceed when the manuscript has been returned with a polite letter of rejection from the managing editor? The first thing to do is to determine the nature of the rejection. Has the article been totally rejected or is there still an opportunity to re-submit after appropriate modification? Clearly it is extremely important to read the editor's rejection letter carefully. This may involve elements of 'reading between the lines' because you may have to determine whether or not rejection has occurred because of such factors as 'salami slicing' or inadvertent or deliberate product sponsorship, rather than experimental design or data analysis. Editors welcome the opportunity to view previous publications on the same subject from authors if there is any suggestion of salami slicing. The prudent author will pre-empt the risk of such an accusation by including reprints of any such material with the original manuscript submission. If the article has been irrevocably rejected by the journal then the editor's letter will say so and may well indicate the reasons. If this is the case, then further communication in the hope of precipitating a dialogue through which you hope to persuade the editors to change their decision will invariably prove ineffective. The time is much better spent by careful examination of the reviewer's criticisms with the aim of responding to the comments and improving the manuscript prior to submission to an alternative journal. Even when the referees' comments appear to be supportive it should be appreciated that the editors' final decision results from a synthesis of two or more reviewer's critiques (which you should receive) together with each referee's structured assessment (which you will not receive) of such factors as originality, timeliness, study design, analysis of results, statistics and conclusions. There may even be factors such as pressure on space in the journal which may weigh in the balance for an editor's decision against acceptance. Editors will rarely reverse a decision for outright rejection no matter how powerful the arguments for reconsideration might appear to the authors.

A further good reason for careful reading of the rejection letter is that it might include an invitation to resubmit a modified version of the manuscript after responding to the criticisms of the referees. Such an invitation does not imply that the re-submitted manuscript will automatically be accepted for publication. Such resubmissions are carefully scrutinised for appropriate modifications and most journals place a time-limit (usually 2 or 3 months), after which any resubmission will be treated as a new submission. It may occasionally appear that requests from the managing editor (for example a request to shorten the manuscript) conflict with a suggestion by the referee (e.g. to expand the discussion to make additional points). Under such circumstances if both instructions can be accommodated well and good, but remember that requests from the editors are likely to take precedence because they have to take into consideration the overall balance of the journal. If the editor suggests that the article is far too long for the message it has to transmit and recommends shortening each section by a certain percentage then you should do so. Failure to respond to the editor's requests will certainly jeopardise the chances of success of any resubmission.

Resubmission

If there is an invitation to resubmit a manuscript the referees' criticisms will clearly have to be addressed and a letter indicating where this has occurred should accompany the revised manuscript. It is prudent to assume that the resubmission will be re-refereed although this is not always the case if the criticisms are of a relatively minor nature. In general each itemised comment should be answered even if in your view there are cogent reasons why the criticism may be irrelevant. Certainly you will need to provide very good reasons for not responding to a particular referee's comment if it is not intended to change the manuscript on this point. It then becomes a matter for the individual editor to determine whether or not a particular criticism can be ignored; this may well involve a further critical opinion before a final decision is reached about publication. The more additional referees that are brought into play, the more questions will be raised about the acceptability of the manuscript. Editors greatly value expert referees and are more likely to accept their advice about publication of a manuscript than opinions implied by the authors. Above all do not assume that addressing all the comments to your satisfaction will guarantee that the article will be accepted. In particular you should under no circumstances refer to the article as being 'in press' until you have received the letter confirming acceptance for publication.

Do not be argumentative

The nature of the criticisms provided by the referees requires careful attention. The review process always improves a manuscript even where there is disagreement with the referee's opinions. Comments about style and presentation are readily dealt with, as are suggestions for further statistical analysis of the data reported in the original manuscript. An invitation to resubmit a manuscript after responding to the referee's comments should also be regarded as an opportunity to confirm that the manuscript conforms to the house style and instructions to authors and does not breach copyright. It is much more difficult to respond to conceptual criticisms and those which relate to experimental design once a particular series of experiments or clinical studies have been completed and it is no longer possible to return to the original laboratory technology or experimental set-up. Fundamental criticisms of the study design which would mean repeating experiments or revisiting the clinical scenario are particularly difficult to handle. A value judgement will have to be made on whether it is worthwhile re-submitting the article (if invited to do so) or simply submitting to a possibly less influential journal after incorporating a suitable comment into the manuscript which acknowledges the weakness of the study, but explains the rationale for undertaking it in the manner described. This decision is a difficult one to reach and requires skill and experience. Junior authors are well advised to work closely with more experienced colleagues within a particular field in order to optimise the chances of a successful resubmission. Criticisms about the conclusions reached from a given data set are again relatively straightforward to respond to, except where there are fundamental differences of opinion about the interpretation between the authors and the referees. It is then a matter of judgement on the part of the senior author to decide whether or not it is worth arguing the point with the editors in the case of an invited resubmission to the original journal, or whether on a point of principle the article should be submitted to a different journal with the original interpretation intact. The latter is relatively unusual because a balanced view is generally possible and enables a response to be generated which, with careful crafting, is acceptable to all parties. Again, an experienced senior view is invaluable.

Value the referees' reports

The reviewers' comments are of great value to an author even when a journal has rejected an article without inviting a resubmission. They provide a steer to improving the manuscript for submission to another journal and it is not unknown for the same referee to be asked to provide an opinion on a paper submitted to a second journal following rejection by the first. Accordingly, where possible, and without prolonging the manuscript, it is useful to pre-empt a repetition of the first reviewer's criticisms by somehow incorporating them into the text of the new manuscript. When the rejected article has been returned, if it is to be resubmitted to an alternative journal then this should be done as soon as possible. Clinical science has a relatively short half-life and the sooner the article is in print the better. Whether or not the paper should be submitted to a journal which has a lower impact factor than the one to which it was originally submitted is a matter of individual judgement. A decision to send it to a higher impact factor journal is risky because the chances of rejection will be correspondingly higher and this will inevitably incur delay in final publication. The choice of journal involves a consideration not only of impact factors but degree of specialisation and other factors. It is important for authors to seek advice from others in the field as to the appropriateness or otherwise of a particular journal for a specific manuscript. Chapter 3 advises on where to send your manuscript. When modifying the manuscript for submission to a different journal it is absolutely critical to ensure that the new version is in the correct house style for that journal. Editors take an understandable dislike to manuscripts submitted in a format which is very obviously that of a competitor journal, even though they appreciate that such resubmissions occur commonly. Failure to adopt the correct house style of a journal gives an impression of imprecision and sloppiness on the part of the author which is unacceptable to editors.

Conclusion

The editors' letter of rejection and the copies of the referees' critiques contain important pointers to the re-writing of a rejected manuscript in a form which may make it acceptable for re-submission either to the original journal or to an alternative one if the rejection is irrevocable. Considerable skill and experience will be required to construct a suitable response to certain criticisms of design and suggestions of flawed experimentation which for practical reasons cannot be revisited. Under these circumstances the advice of senior colleagues who have a feel for the journals' expectations, and reactions to what may be challenging conflicts of opinion are invaluable. If the manuscript is to be resubmitted to the original journal or elsewhere, then do so promptly. Be reassured that the majority of articles are published somewhere eventually, but the longer you temporise, the lower are the chances of publication. Remember that each submission-rejection cycle may take from 3 to 6 months. Be resolved and persistent and you will get there eventually. However, do not lose sight of the aims of publication which are both educational and serve to disseminate new knowledge which may, directly or indirectly, influence clinical practice. Selection of the appropriate journal for the first submission is almost as important in avoiding rejection as having the idea and undertaking the research in the first place!

Commentary
by R. E. Condon
Professor and Chairman, Emeritus, Department of Surgery, The Medical College of Wisconsin, Milwaukee, U.S.A.

For a neophyte surgical author, the most difficult experience related to publishing is dealing with rejection. You've done your best and have been turned down. Disheartening! The best thing to do in this circumstance is to remember the song line, 'pick yourself up and get back in the race.' Persistence pays and those who keep at it eventually get their article published.

In reviewing reasons for rejection, case reports have to be considered separately. The typical case report is offered for publication because the disease, clinical setting, or other circumstances are rare or unusual. Such reports are regularly rejected, even by those few journals that still accept them. The only reason to publish a case report is that it contains a new, useful and generalizable insight into diagnosis or treatment. Rarity is not a reason. Don't waste further time and effort unless it embodies or illustrates something truly novel and indispensable.

In preparing and submitting most types of articles to professional journals, the advice in this chapter is cogent and should be heeded. Objective evaluation of the worth of your article and a good choice in matching the

191

content of your report to the interests of the readers of a journal are essential steps but rejection still occurs. Rejection is not always a judgment by the Editor that the article is unworthy. There are numerous reasons for rejection.

Editors try to keep the delay from acceptance to publication reasonably short, so you may have been turned down only because the queue of articles awaiting publication is too long. The journal may have recently accepted an article by another author reporting similar findings and conclusions. The Editor may not want repetitive publication. You may have had the bad luck of having your article assigned to an obtuse and churlish reviewer but pay attention to these messages when revising your manuscript for publication elsewhere.

Finally, remember that there is no more difficult task than getting a truly new idea published. Editors and reviewers are more comfortable with what they already know. The unknown is a different matter. The history of medicine and science is replete with stories of the initial rejection of important new ideas. Those authors persisted despite rejection, eventually got published, and we are now the better for it. When a rejection letter arrives consider that you are in the best company; Nobel prize-winners have been rejected! Don't give up; revise and resubmit.

Chapter 19

Research misconduct: diagnosis, treatment and prevention

M. J. G. Farthing

Professor of Medicine

University of Glasgow

Glasgow, UK

Introduction

Research misconduct has probably existed for as long as researchers have researched. The temptation to enhance or embellish a research finding with a few extra experiments that were never done or to trim away 'inconvenient results' have been there as long as man has had a desire to answer scientific questions through experimentation. Even outright fraud is not a new phenomenon with examples going back as far as Mendel's work several centuries ago.

During the past decade, however, research misconduct has been placed firmly in the public eye with increasing coverage of cases by daily newspapers concerning the sacking of academics by universities and a substantial number of disciplinary hearings by the General Medical Council (GMC) [1].

A further indication of the seriousness of the problem is reflected by the development in many countries of agencies to deal with cases of suspected research misconduct such as the Office of Research Integrity in the USA and similar bodies in Scandinavia, other European countries and Australia. Thus, there is the impression that research misconduct in all of its forms is on the increase because of the serendipitous nature of many of the discoveries of misconduct. Many feel that we may be looking at the tip of a rather large iceberg.

I came face to face with publication ethics when I became Editor of *Gut*, a specialist journal for gastroenterology and hepatology [2]. In my first year we detected redundant publication (an attempt to publish data the majority of which had been published in another journal in the preceding year), 'salami slicing' (publishing a study piece meal when a single, high quality paper would have been preferable), outright plagiarism and papers being submitted without the knowledge or consent of co-authors. Compared to the major cases of fraud that have come to light in the last year or so, these are relatively minor offences and all were detected prior to publication. Retractions were not required and no author faced public disgrace. However, they raised important questions for me as the Editor and I hope for the individuals concerned when their actions were discovered. Unlike some countries in the world, the United Kingdom has no regulatory agency which deals with research misconduct, although the most serious cases of overt fraud are reported to the General Medical Council (GMC), which can result in a judgement of serious professional misconduct and removal from the GMC register.

There is a feeling among editors and some investigators that research misconduct has become more frequent during the last two decades. It is difficult to be certain whether this perceived increase is a true increase in the number of misdemeanours committed but there is no doubt that the number of serious cases of research misconduct that have been detected has increased during this period. Stephen Lock, a past editor of the *British Medical Journal* documented known or suspected cases of research misconduct in the UK, USA, Australia, Canada and other countries [1]. In the UK many of the cases involve fabrication of clinical trial data most commonly by general practitioners although hospital clinicians have been guilty of similar offences. Fraud in laboratory experimentation appears less common although there have been a number of notorious cases in the USA and UK when the results of laboratory experiments have been fabricated, falsified or misrepresented.

What is research misconduct?

There are many misdemeanours that are commonly brought together under the headings of research and publication misconduct [3]. At the milder end of the spectrum there are sins of omission; an example would be when experimental design is inadequate to answer the questions raised in the study. Similarly the inappropriate use of statistical analyses may produce inaccuracies both in the final results and in the conclusions reached. This occurs through ignorance but also by intent. Selective presentation of results through data suppression or exclusion may similarly influence the research findings to produce apparently 'clear cut' results but which are at the same time misleading. It is always easier to write a paper when everything fits neatly together! Finally the major offences of fabrication, falsification and plagiarism constitute outright research fraud. It is these major crimes that have been picked up avidly by the daily press and in the UK have resulted in doctors being struck off by the GMC. Some scientists argue that even overtly fraudulent research is not as dangerous as many would like to have us believe, since others will repeat the work and if false, will eventually put the record right and make this clear in the biomedical literature. I would argue that this 'soft line' makes a complete nonsense of the fundamental premise on which scientific research is based, namely 'honesty'. In addition, it is a deplorable waste of time and resources to prove that fraudulent research is false. In addition, damage can be done before the truth about falsified research eventually comes to light as illustrated by a paper published in 1993 in the *British Medical Journal* that was subsequently retracted last year after five years exposure in the public domain. This paper was of sufficient public health importance to change the delivery of services in a region of the United Kingdom.

There are instances when there are no questions about a way in which a piece of research was conducted, but in the process of preparing the manuscript for publication and the manner in which the paper is presented to a journal, the authors commit publication misconduct. A common problem centres on authorship. It is now well recognised that individuals' names often appear on a paper whose contribution to the work is questionable, so-called 'gift authorship'. The Vancouver group of Editors have published guidelines on what constitutes authorship. This would, for example, exclude a widely held custom to include the Head of Department as a 'courtesy' (Table 1) [4]. There is now a move away from authorship but towards contributorship in which each individual outlines at the end of the paper their individual contributions to the work. There would also be a guarantor who would take overall responsibility for the veracity of the paper [5]. Disputes between authors are also common ranging from failure to get approval from all authors before the final manuscript is

TABLE 1
Authorship

Authorship credit should be based only on substantial contributions to:

◇   (a)   Conception and design or analysis and interpretation of data; and to

◇   (b)   Drafting the article or revising it critically for important intellectual content; and on

◇   (c)   Final approval of the version to be published

          Conditions (a), (b) and (c) must all be met.

◇   Participation solely in the acquisition of funding or the collection of data does not justify authorship.

◇   General supervision of the research group is also not sufficient for authorship.

From reference 4

submitted to a journal, to changes in authorship or the order of authors during manuscript revisions.

Some authors still submit papers simultaneously to two journals (dual submission) while others attempt to identify 'the minimal publishable unit' sometimes referred to as 'salami slicing'. Most editors would prefer to see a substantial manuscript containing a cohesive story rather than a string of minor contributions in a variety of different journals.

197

Failure to declare conflicts of interest is another aspect of publication misconduct. Conflicts include direct or indirect financial support from the study, consultancy agreement with a study sponsor, a holding of any patents relating to the study and any other mechanisms by which financial benefits might accrue as a result of publication of the study. It has been said, 'disclosure is almost a panacea'.

Does research misconduct exist in Britain?

In 1988 Stephen Lock, then Editor of the *British Medical Journal*, published a paper in that journal summarising the findings of a survey conducted in twenty-nine medical institutions in Britain from which there were seventy-nine respondents, many of whom were Professors of Medicine and Surgery [6]. More than half knew cases of research misconduct, many of which involved senior academics and only a minority of the cases had been investigated. He concluded that there was a definite problem in Britain and that the results of this survey were likely to be an underestimate.

During the past five years there have been a number of major fraud cases that have been drawn to the public's attention and during the last two years the GMC has received thirty-one complaints relating to alleged drug trial misconduct or fraud. The size of the problem in the UK remains completely unknown as current impressions rely entirely on the detected misdemeanours.

Who are the fraudsters?

Research misconduct has been committed across the age-experience spectrum. Fabrication of clinical trial data, usually the addition of fictitious patients to a randomised controlled trial, may involve a relatively naïve, inexperienced investigator such as the general practitioner or a senior hospital consultant [1]. In some instances the motivation is financial, driven by the knowledge that the more patients recruited to the study, the greater the rewards. Studies driven by the pharmaceutical industry are usually closely monitored such that detection of research fraud becomes evident when clinical report forms cannot be matched to patients' clinical records. Sometimes fraudulent clinical investigators will persuade research associates to collude with the fraudulent process.

Another category of fraudster is the young laboratory scientist who succumbs to the pressure for academic success and promotion and the institutional demands to secure research funding. These individuals are often medically qualified, male and working in a distinguished institution within a productive research group. The individual almost invariably has a list of publications that is growing at a rate well beyond that normally expected from someone at that stage in their career. Research data may be fabricated completely or falsified by selected deletion and/or supplementation. Other laboratory colleagues often suspect that such a person is working in a dishonest way but are generally disinclined to come forward as the 'whistle blower'.

Research and publication dishonesty crosses all age groups, disciplines and levels of seniority.

Diagnosis

Serious research fraud is usually discovered during the formal audit or monitoring process of randomised controlled trials when all patients apparently recruited into the study cannot be accounted for from a search of independent medical records. Fraudulent clinical trials have also been detected after publication, often when there are some unusual features to the study. Surprising, unexpected results emerging from an apparently, large single-centre study written up by a single author might attract attention. Published work may come into question when an investigator is found to have committed research misconduct and then previously published fraudulent work is then revealed following a systematic review of the contents of the author's curriculum vitae. The other important route by which research fraud is detected is through a 'whistle blower', commonly a colleague in the same or a closely related department. Although there are many examples when 'whistle blowers' have subsequently suffered more than the accused there is now a firm legal framework to protect people in the workplace who become concerned about the behaviour of colleagues.

One of the most active, contemporary 'whistle blowers' in the UK is Peter Wilmshurst, a consultant cardiologist in Shrewsbury. Wilmshurst wrote an article in *The Lancet* in 1997 entitled 'The code of silence' in which he suggested that there were a number of cases of research misconduct in the UK that had not been adequately investigated or suppressed, perhaps by senior members of the profession [7]. One of the cases referred to anonymously in this report was finally brought before the Professional Conduct Committee of the GMC in November 2000 and resulted in the suspension of Dr Anjan Banerjee, a surgeon from Halifax [8,9]. It took almost a decade for this case to be resolved despite the fact that many colleagues knew of the allegations for much of this period. Certain individuals who had been willing to speak out were silenced with the threat that their future career would be at stake. Peter Wilmshurst assembled the evidence and eventually the case was heard. Without his tenacity it is unlikely that Banerjee would have been required to face his misdemeanours nor would the medical literature have been corrected.

This sounds like a satisfactory ending to an otherwise sad story. However a number of issues remain unresolved. As editor of the journal in which Banerjee published his fraudulent work, I am responsible for issuing a retraction notice in the journal, a request which came promptly from the author following the GMC judgement. However it is extremely difficult to effectively erase an article from the published literature since the November 1990 issue of *Gut* will remain on library shelves for many decades to come without any indication that the Banerjee paper is fraudulent. In addition we know that retracted papers continue to be cited after retraction almost invariably without reference to the falsehoods that are contained therein [10]. If publication of scientific material becomes solely electronic, only then will it be possible to completely erase a paper and put the record straight. Another issue is the delay that has occurred in bringing this case to the GMC. Intuitively most of us would believe that it would be preferable to solve a crime promptly to minimise the risk that further misdemeanours might be committed. Banerjee had already been suspended by his NHS Trust and is awaiting a further hearing at the GMC. Whether earlier resolution of the research misconduct case would have influenced this issue remains a matter for speculation.

Unfortunately the case does not rest here. Banerjee's supervisor at the time he produced the fraudulent work, Professor Tim Peters, subsequently also appeared before the GMC, and was found guilty of serious professional misconduct; he was given a severe reprimand. Finally, and perhaps most important of all, will be to determine what happened following the earlier internal enquiry of the Banerjee case at King's College Hospital Medical School. If Banerjee's work, as it is alleged, was found to be questionable at that time [7], why did the Dean of the day not refer the case to the GMC immediately? Why was the *Gut* paper not retracted in 1991 and why did Banerjee's supervisor remain associated with the work when other collaborators withdrew their names from the paper? It is likely that answers to all or some of these questions will come out of subsequent GMC hearings.

We all have a responsibility to be vigilant about the quality of research with which we are directly or indirectly associated. If you have suspicions that a colleague may be producing research findings dishonestly, the most important first step is to ensure that you obtain evidence of your suspicions before reporting this to a senior colleague. In some instances it may be entirely appropriate to discuss this with the person concerned particularly if you feel that the main problem is 'trimming and pruning' which the individual may be pursuing out of ignorance. Similarly, if there are potential misdemeanours regarding publication ethics such as dual submission or redundant publication then these should be dealt with by open discussion. However, if the misdemeanours are of a more serious nature such as fabrication or falsification of research data then you must be able to provide evidence of the misdemeanours before reporting to a higher authority. Potential 'whistle blowers' may have to wait weeks or even months to ensure that their suspicions are well founded. At this point discussions should occur with the head of department, although if that individual is directly involved with the research it may be more appropriate to discuss concerns immediately with the head of the institution. At this point a preliminary enquiry should be performed along the lines described in the Royal College of Physicians Working Party Report [11] or as described in the Medical Research Council's document which describes a procedure for enquiring into allegations of scientific misconduct within MRC units [12].

Journal editors and reviewers also detect research and publication misconduct. As an editor of a specialist journal, sharp-eyed reviewers have drawn my attention to the majority of cases of misconduct in the past three years. However, in almost every case there has been an element of serendipity about the discovery. For example, in one case of plagiarism, I just happened, by chance, to send the manuscript to a reviewer whose papers had been plagiarised. How many other manuscripts have passed through the system and escaped detection because the reviewer did not have such an intimate knowledge of the text of related papers? Redundant publication and 'salami slicing' is again usually detected by expert reviewers who know their subject well. On several occasions, a manuscript goes, by chance, to a reviewer who has been sent a closely related and in some cases identical manuscript by the same authors from another journal, simultaneously. In this case publication can be stopped. If the manuscript had been sent to another reviewer, who had not seen the closely related manuscript, then both manuscripts could have entered the public domain with inevitable redundancy. The detection of publication and research misconduct seems to carry with it a large element of chance and many editors of biomedical journals suspect that only a small proportion of misdemeanours are detected. It would appear that crime does pay! Diagnostic approaches would thus, seem to be inadequate and given the obvious limitations that a 'whistle blower', editor or reviewer might have perhaps we should focus our attention more on treatment and prevention.

Treatment

When serious fraud, such as fabrication of controlled clinical trial data, is detected, the person or persons concerned would be reported to the GMC. If a preliminary review of the evidence suggests that there were sufficient grounds to proceed, then the GMC would hold a full enquiry and if the defendant is found guilty this might result in exclusion from the Medical Register. For lesser crimes and those involving non-clinical scientists, a 'whistle blower' or journal editor might refer the case to the Head of the investigator's department or institution. Reporting an individual to the Head of institution, however, may not necessarily produce a satisfactory outcome, as there may be conflict of interest. For example, the senior author might be a prominent clinical academic within the institution and possibly even a personal friend of the Dean or Vice-chancellor. There are a number of instances of alleged, serious research misconduct that have been 'silenced' within the investigator's institution. It is difficult to feel confident that internal enquiries into alleged research misconduct held 'in camera' will reliably get at the truth when for the institution there is so much to lose and little to gain.

Editors face some difficult issues when they suspect or detect research fraud. Once a journal has published a paper that is subsequently shown to be fraudulent or redundant then the paper would be retracted and a notice to that effect published in the journal. This places the case in the public domain and the authors are exposed. In serious cases the editor may, in the case of clinical investigators, refer the matter to the GMC. A recent study has shown, however, that this does not stop the paper being cited in the literature for many years, usually without making any reference to the fabrication or falsification contained therein [10].

It is however, more difficult to know precisely how to act when research misconduct is suspected during the peer review process before publication. The most common editorial response is to simply reject the manuscript. This is clearly unsatisfactory and one might argue that the editor has not fulfilled a duty as a custodian of the biomedical literature since it is likely that the paper would merely be submitted to another journal. Some editors have taken a 'hard line' and have placed sanctions on all authors who engage in redundant publication, such as refusing to accept further submissions to the journal for a set period, say three years [13]. Editors who are members of the Committee for Publication Ethics [14] (COPE) have produced some guidelines on *Good Publication Practice* (see Appendix I. Also available in the 1999 COPE Report [15] or on the COPE website www.publicationethics.org.UK) which set down a hierarchy of sanctions which editors may publish in journals and use judiciously such that 'the punishment fits the crime'. These might range from a firm letter to the author pointing out the breach of publication ethics when it is felt that an error occurred through ignorance and not mal-intent, to tougher sanctions such as limited access to the journal for a given period as described above or ultimately to referral of the matter to the author's head of institution or directly to the GMC. The Royal College of Physicians, London and the MRC have produced guidance on the investigation and prevention of research misconduct [11,12].

Prevention

Investigators may be less inclined to commit research and publication misconduct if they knew the chances of getting caught and punished were increased. Ultimately however, the route to prevention must be through education and reaffirmation of the still widely held belief in the principle of research honesty. All students entering a period of research should receive instruction on research design, methodology and laboratory techniques but also guidance on the fundamentals of research and publication ethics (Table 2). Research should be protocol driven and contributors and collaborators should define their roles before the work is commenced. Any protocol changes should be discussed and agreed by all of the participants. Statistical advice should be sought, where appropriate, during the planning process and it goes without saying that all studies involving human subjects should be submitted to an appropriate research ethics committee. There is a sense that at least some of the instances of research misconduct could have been avoided by closer supervision of the project. Supervisors can find themselves increasingly distanced from the laboratory bench or the patients in the clinic, which can make it difficult to check the veracity of the primary data. Review of research results should involve examination of the primary research record that may be the laboratory record book or patients' medical notes. Impeccable record keeping is an essential component of good research.

The ethics of publication is as important as research ethics. All authors should see the final manuscript before submission and each sign the declaration confirming the originality of the work. An article should only be submitted to one journal at a time. Authors should disclose any potential conflicts of interest particularly if the opinions expressed in the manuscript could be influenced by financial incentives through sponsors. Authors should also disclose the nature of any related publications that have been published recently or that are under consideration by another journal. There are times when it is entirely reasonable to publish some previously published data but this should be done with the full knowledge of the editor and reviewers enabling a full assessment of the extent of any potential overlap. In the future, original research may be submitted to random audit prior to publication and it is, therefore, wise that authors assume that they may be asked to produce primary data to support the work described in a manuscript.

TABLE 2
Prevention of research and publication misconduct

Education

Research training
Research ethics
Publication ethics

The research

Protocol driven
Establish contributors & collaborators

Define roles
Agree protocol
Agree presentation of results

Define methodology for data analysis
Ethical approval
Project and personal licence (Home Office)
Supervision

Statistical advice

Guarantor
Communication
Ensure Good Clinical Practice
Record keeping

The publication

Disclose conflict of interest
Disclose previous publication
Approval by **all** contributors
Submit to one journal at a time
Assume research data audit

The future

The recent Banerjee case at the GMC illustrates a number of important deficiencies in the way in which we handle possible cases of research misconduct in the UK. Firstly, it is evident that it is relatively simple to fabricate data and get it published in a reputable medical journal. In the majority of cases it will be virtually impossible for reviewers and editors to identify fraudulent material. Detection in this case, and in many others will almost always depend on the willingness of a vigilant 'whistle blower' to speak out. As stated previously, there is little in it for the 'whistle blower', particularly when their comments fall on 'deaf ears' or they are threatened with professional extinction. Secondly, the case demonstrates the potential weakness of the internal enquiry. Although it is unclear as to the location of the final resting place of the King's Banerjee Report, it is alleged that its findings were not in Banerjee's favour [7]. It then took almost a decade and the persistent efforts of an external 'whistle blower' who had no conflicting interests to bring the case to the GMC. This cannot be regarded as a satisfactory state of affairs and will do nothing to reassure the public that the medical profession is still fit to self regulate. The case also shows the importance of the role of the research supervisor as a custodian of research quality. When it was clear in 1991 that Banerjee's work was suspect, why did he not withdraw his support and insist on an external review by the GMC?

This case, others considered by COPE, and probably others still in the GMC pipeline, convince me that the procedures currently in place in the UK are inadequate to deal with many of the possible instances of research misconduct. COPE has campaigned for more than three years for an independent body to consider such cases [16]. Although many Universities and Medical Schools have written guidance as to how to pursue an internal review, I have concerns that a lack of independence may not be facilitatory for an otherwise reluctant 'whistle blower' and provide appropriate protection when required. In October 1999 a consensus conference was held at the Royal College of Physicians in Edinburgh on Misconduct in Biomedical Research. The consensus panel recommended that a National Panel should be established which would develop and promote models of good practice for local implementation, provide assistance with the investigation of alleged research misconduct, and collect, collate and publish information on the incidence of research misconduct. Although discussions have taken place and a report is said to be in preparation, no clear action has yet become apparent [9,17]. Even if such an advisory panel is established will it really have the teeth to ensure that we do not have a re-run of the Banerjee case? I have my doubts. What COPE is proposing is not new. The USA, Nordic countries and others have had external agencies in place to deal with alleged cases of research misconduct for almost 10 years [18]; why is the UK lagging behind? One is reminded of the fact that it took 20 years longer to establish Research Ethics Committees in Britain than it did in the USA!

References

1   Lock S. Research misconduct: a résumé of recent events. In, *Fraud and misconduct in medical research.* Ed. S. Lock, F. Wells. 2nd Edition BMJ Publishing Group, London 1996, pp 14-39.

2   Farthing MJG. Research misconduct. *Gut* 1997; 41: 1-2

3   Farthing MJG. Ethics of Publication. In, *How to write a paper.* Ed. G.M. Hall. 2nd Edition. BMJ Books, London 1998.

4   International Committee of Medical Journal Editors. Uniform requirements for manuscripts submitted to biomedical journals. *Ann Intern Med* 1997; 126: 36-47.

5   Smith R. Authorship: time for a paradigm shift? *BMJ* 1997; 314: 992.

6   Lock S. Misconduct in medical research: Does it exist in Britain? *BMJ* 1988; 297: 1531-535.

7   Wilmshurst P. The code of silence. *Lancet* 1997; 349: 567-69

8   Ferriman A. Consultant suspended for research fraud. *BMJ* 2000; 321: 1429

9   White C. Plans for tackling research fraud may not go far enough. *BMJ* 2000; 321: 1487

10 Budd JM, Sievert ME, Schultz TR. Phenomena of retraction. *JAMA* 1998; 280: 296-297.

11 Working Party. Fraud and misconduct in medical research. Causes, investigation and prevention. Royal College of Physicians, London 1991.

12 Medical Research Council. Policy and procedure for inquiring into allegations of scientific misconduct. MRC Ethics Series, December 1997. Aldridge Print Group, Surrey.

13 Doherty M. The misconduct of redundant publication. *Ann Rheum Dis* 1996; 55: 783-5.

14 The COPE (Committee on Publication Ethics) Report 1998. Eds A. Williamson, C. White. BMJ Publishing Group, London 1998.

15 The COPE Report 1999. Annual Report of the Committee on Publication Ethics. Ed C. White. BMJ Books, London 1999

16 Farthing MJG. An editor's response to fraudsters. *BMJ* 1998; 316: 1729-31

17 Farthing M, Horton R, Smith R. UK's failure to act on research misconduct. *Lancet* 2000; 356: 2030

18 Nylenna M, Andersen D, Dahlquist G, Sarvas M, Aakvaag. Handling of scientific dishonesty in the Nordic countries. *Lancet* 1999; 354: 57-61

Commentary
by G. M. Stirrat

Emeritus Professor of Obstetrics & Gynaecology, and Senior Research Fellow in Ethics in Medicine, Centre for Ethics in Medicine, University of Bristol, Bristol, UK.

'Research - Investigation or experimentation aimed at the discovery and interpretation of facts, revision of accepted theories or laws in the light of new facts or practical application of such new or revised theories or laws' [1]. Thus, a word trail starting with 'research' soon brings us to 'facts' and then to 'truth'. The concept of truth and the honest search for it are deeply unfashionable in this post-modernist world that denies the possibility of neutral or objective thought [2]. In my opinion, the erosion *of the Kantian concept of scientific or a posteriori truth [7] derived from experience based knowledge and empirical research has removed a vital standard from our individual and collective discipline. If truth cannot be found who is to say what un-truth is?*

In 1992, Arnold [4] wrote 'Like politics, the sciences operate on the basis of control, operant conditioning (rule by carrot and stick), stimulus/response, input/output and a pre-occupation with symptoms and operations. As a result most scientists play a mechanistic, quantitatively competitive (winning and losing) rather than qualitatively competitive (co-operative and organic) game'. One of the consequences is that subsidiary objectives dominate our research. Among them are adding to one's curriculum vitae and responding to the demands of the Research Assessment Exercise and analogous processes in the National Health Service in the UK and other countries. Thus process has <u>become</u> purpose rather than being its servant. The pressure to obtain grants and publish papers as ends in themselves, in a climate in which the concept of scientific truth is belittled, inevitably increases the temptation to indulge in research misconduct as described by Farthing [5]. Another aspect not often considered is the risk that those undertaking peer review of grant applications and papers obtain personal advantage by 'doing down' those working in the same field as themselves.

In his scheme to prevent research misconduct, Farthing [5] correctly emphasises the need to reaffirm the principle of research honesty and suggests beginning a process of education when students commence research. The merit of this proposal is that it is something that we can actually do. However, given that the way we carry out our research directly reflects the ethics of the society in which we live, those ethical principles must be much more widely discussed in society and inculcated from early in the curricula of our schools. In the often quoted phrase from John Donne [6] 'No man is an island entire of it self (sic); every man is a piece of the Continent, a part of the main'.

References

1   *Merriam Webster Collegiate Dictionary.* Encyclopaedia Britannica, 1999.

2   Ermath ED (2000). Postmodernism. *Concise Routledge Encylcopaedia of Philosophy.* Routledge, London, pp699-700.

3   Kant I (1781/1787). *Critique of Pure Reason translated by N. Kemp Smith.* Macmillan, London, 1963.

4   Arnold A (1992). *The Corrupted Sciences.* Paladin, London, p37.

5   Farthing MJG (2001). Research Misconduct: diagnosis, treatment and prevention. In *'A surgeon's guide to writing and publishing'.* Eds Schein, Farndon and Fingerhut.

6   Donne J (1624). Devotions upon Emerg.

Chapter
19

Chapter 20

Internet communication and e-publishing

W. D. Neary

Vascular Research Fellow,
Gloucestershire Royal Hospital
Gloucester, UK

J. J. Earnshaw

Consultant Surgeon,
Gloucestershire Royal Hospital
Gloucester, UK

Introduction

Future generations may acknowledge that mass publishing really began with the Internet revolution rather than with Caxton's printing press. This massive increase in the availability of knowledge has implications for surgeon scientists wishing to spread information; for publishers of paper journals and books; and for clinicians seeking information on which to base a modern, evidence-based approach to surgical practice. Attitudes have to be established in surgeons and publishers to optimize the delivery of surgical knowledge. The most influential providers of information in the future will be those who create the best balance. The challenge is to harness the immense power of the Internet in a way that is usable, while maintaining a role for books and journals for those who prefer them.

Advantages and disadvantages of e-publishing

For almost the whole of the twentieth century the peer-review system held sway for the refereeing of scientific information before publication. In peer-review, supposed unbiased referees check a scientific article sent to a journal before publication. Despite much research, there is no significant alternative to this system [1,2]. With electronic publication, it is possible for anyone to post research on an Internet site at any time without restriction. This does have the advantage of immediacy and scientific advances can be brought into the public arena instantly and disseminated widely. This suits some scientific writers more than others. It also appeals to popular opinion; society abhors secrecy and delay, wishing to be aware of advances as soon as possible. Some scientific writers feel that the peer review system is unfair, and it can be slow and cumbersome. In some journals it can take a year or more from submission of an article to publication.

Peer review has, however, stood the test of time. Journals which use it collect articles of a certain standard into a single medium (the issues of the journal) where surgeons can read approved knowledge and information. Most recognise that peer review provides a stamp of approval to published information. Whether or not an article is published, independent peer review often helps to improve the content or quality of a scientific manuscript.

Removing the barriers to surgical publishing by abolishing the hurdle of peer review could open Pandora's Box. Without control, quantities of unmonitored information could be posted on the World Wide Web, diluting and hiding quality research. It could be argued that surgeons and scientists should be able to assess the quality of information themselves but non-surgeons have access to the web and may not be so discerning. In such an open system it could be difficult to find high quality information.

Electronic publication could broaden access to surgical information. Whereas journals and books may not penetrate much of Africa and Eastern block countries, access to the Internet could be universal. European governments have expressed a wish to extend processing power to developing nations but equipment is expensive and rapidly becomes obsolete.

Possible solutions

One solution is to adapt the peer review process for the electronic era and make it more open. The *British Medical Journal* [3] and the *New England Journal of Medicine* have pioneered the response of existing weekly journals with the development of on-line correspondence columns. Submitted letters are placed onto Journal web sites and left for open peer review, publication in the journal depends on the responses received. Approximately 15% of letters posted on the *BMJ* rapid response site are published in the paper Journal [3].

This brings into question the value of publication in a Journal. Surgeons publish for two reasons - to further science and to enhance their own careers. Journal publication results in a reference on a curriculum vitae. It remains to be decided how e-publication can be accredited and whether the reference is as valuable.

An alternative solution is to gather all scientific medical writing into a single site with open electronic peer review: Biomed Central is an attempt at this. The concept is that unlike publication in a journal, a piece of scientific research is dynamic and may be changed, upgraded, revisited or even retracted over time. Comment and criticism can be pooled. Publication in a citable journal can follow, without prejudice.

Publishing in conventional surgical journals could be speeded up by using a system of electronic submission and manuscript handling. Software is now available to enable the entire process of manuscript submission, refereeing and editing without resort to paper copy. Several scientific journals are now published entirely in an electronic format [4] and subscribers have to read articles from a computer screen. Many people find this uncomfortable, though it may be easier with the new generation of flat screen monitors. A paper copy is technically no further away than the printer button but piles of paper compare poorly with a professionally bound journal. The future is likely to see a combination of both: a rapid publication electronic journal (preprints or eprints) with a subsequent paper journal for ease of reading.

The funding of electronic journals will be a major issue. Publishers currently rely on subscriptions. Open availability of information on the Internet is good for readers but reduces the value of subscription to a journal. There is a danger that publishers will go out of business or lose interest because of lack of potential profit. There have been similar worries in the music industry. Early observation refutes this, however, and the ability to download music has not reduced sales of compact discs. People who download music are more likely to subsequently purchase the same music on compact disc. Many different industries are actively looking at ways to make money from electronic sites, including websites. Few have yet achieved this.

Doctors will pay for a useful product and a well-maintained electronic site with good links especially if this offers more than just regular access to recent scientific articles. Huge sites such as PubMed Central gather from many different journals and an increasing number are available as full text on-line [5].

The quality of information that has not undergone peer review has been likened to preliminary data presented at a scientific meeting. If members of an audience feel strongly about a presentation, individuals can respond and challenge the author. This facility is mirrored on the Internet by *BMJ* Netprints where unpublished research can be evaluated on-line and comments fed back to the authors. The process is entirely open and can be accessed by professionals and lay persons alike [6].

The evolution of websites and portals

Most editors and publishers have developed a first generation website to highlight and enhance a particular journal. The quality varied hugely and the first and simplest sites offered only subscription details and were maintained by publishers only. Some sites set up by enthusiasts have been left fallow as the burden of maintenance became apparent. To be competitive, a successful journal website must add value over and above the paper issue. Subsequent sites that are managed more actively are evolving. Information and links need to be updated frequently and consequently they are expensive to maintain and potentially loss-making to a journal or publisher.

As second-generation sites grow and accumulate facilities, they have been termed portals [4]. Portals are areas of interconnected information that appeal to single interest groups. A surgeon could, for example, access a journal and on the same website find useful information such as forthcoming conferences, venues and registration details. Distance learning may play a significant part in continuing medical education at all levels and a surgical portal would be a logical place to accumulate such resources. For example, it might be possible to view an overseas conference on a personal computer.

Sites such as Biomednet, or the latest National electronic Library for Health [7], have search engines to databases such as Medline, EM base and the Cochrane library (see Table 1 for electronic addresses). They have links to medical journals and links to groups of articles that may be relevant to a researcher. Links can be customized and may even be subscription-based. A good search engine such as the one that covers the National Library of Medicine database (which has been endorsed by the Royal College of Surgeons) is invaluable. It allows the user to look for specific publication types, for example randomized clinical trials or case reports and permits the user to focus on required information. The Royal College of Surgeons has an electronic site dedicated to evidence based medicine [8].

Exchange of information can be dynamic allowing interaction between surgeons. The Internet has spawned a large number of chat rooms, where individuals swap messages. A portal that recruited surgeons with a shared interest could allow intercommunication either in real time or via e-mail. An e-mail group such as Surginet [9] functions as a large and international forum in which surgeons discuss anything to do with surgical practise, research and teaching (to join SURGINET send an email to: mschein1@mindspring.com). E-groups allow dissemination of information and meeting dates. Surgical trainees have embraced e-groups as an ideal means of informing a group about teaching sessions and local meetings. A good example is the Rouleaux Club, a forum for trainees in vascular surgery in the United Kingdom.

Surgical research: trial registration

The Internet can facilitate surgical research by registering and monitoring clinical trials [10,11]. Registering trial protocols enables widespread constructive criticism at the pretrial stage and can foster

TABLE 1
Useful website addresses

Biomed Central **http://www.biomedcentral.com**

Pubmed Central **http://www.pubmedcentral.nih.gov**

Biomed Net **http://www.bmn.com**

National electronic Library for Health (prototype) **http://www.nelh.nhs.uk**

Cochrane Collaboration **http://www.cochrane.co.uk**

National Library of Medicine **http://www.nlm.nih.gov**

Current controlled trials **http://www.controlled-trials.com**

Royal College of Surgeons of Edinburgh **http://www.rcsed.ac.uk**

Royal College of Surgeons of England **http://www.rcseng.ac.uk**

The Lancet **http://www.thelancet.com/**

New England Journal of Medicine **http://www.nejm.org**

BMJ **http://www.bmj.com** (including Netprints)

British Journal of Surgery **http://www.bjs.co.uk**

Rouleaux Club **http://www.rouleaux.org**

collaboration between groups. Review of existing registers can expose gaps in surgical knowledge that are not currently being explored. Registration may also allow recognition of subsequent publication bias when trials with negative or disappointing findings are not published thereby affecting the process of meta-analysis. The *Lancet* encourages the registration of trial protocols with the offer of subsequent publication if the research reaches fruition.

Conclusions

The electronic revolution offers much to publishers by driving down the cost of journal publication. Electronic journals and their portals must be commercially viable if, as expected, subscriptions to paper journals diminish. Viable sites may need to seek advertising revenue from paper and electronic journals. The existence of a well-defined target audience should help generate interest from advertisers.

Journals that survive the transition to this near unlimited access to information will need a strong electronic presence that adds value to paper copy. As the quantity of information increases, a balance between quality and overload must be found, probably by the development of a robust and accurate electronic search engine. The successful search engines of the future must be able to recognise quality information, probably without recourse to peer review in its current form. Peer review remains unchallenged but could be accelerated using modern electronic communication techniques.

The exciting challenge for the future is how to manage surgical knowledge effectively while allowing equal access to all doctors (and perhaps patients) to high quality information of relevance [12].

References

1   Smith R. Peer review: reform or revolution? *BMJ* 1997; 315: 759-60

2   Godlee F, Jefferson T. *Peer review in health sciences.* BMA Publishing, London 1999.

3   Smith R. Opening up BMJ peer review. *BMJ* 1999; 318: 4-5.

4   Lindsay LA. Information access for the new millenium: publishers and portals. *J R Coll Surg Edinb* 2000; 45: 60-1.

5   Delamothe T, Smith R. PubMed Central: creating an Aladdin's cage of ideas. *BMJ* 2001; 322: 1-2.

6   Delamothe T, Smith R, Keller MA, Sack J, Witscher B. Netprints: the next phase in the evolution of biomedical publishing. *BMJ* 1999; 319: 1515-16.

7   Muir Gray JA, De Lusigan S. National electronic Library for Health (NeLH). *BMJ* 1999; 319: 1476-9.

8   Liu D. Evidence-based surgery and the internet. *Ann R Coll Surg Eng* (suppl) 1999; 81: 115-7.

9   Gilas T, Schein M, Fryberg E. A surgical Internet discussion list (surginet): a novel venue for communication among surgeons. *Arch Surg* 1998: 133; 1126-30.

10   Horton R, Smith R. Time to register randomised trials. *Lancet* 1999; 354: 1138-9.

11   Tonks A. Registering clinical trials. *BMJ* 1999; 319: 1565-8.

12   Muir Gray JA. Where's the chief knowledge officer? *BMJ* 1998; 317: 832-4.

Commentary
by Dr. R. Smith
Editor, BMJ and Chief Executive of the BMJ Publishing Group
BMJ editorial, London, UK

Doctors suffer from the 'information paradox': they are overwhelmed with information, much of it of poor quality, and yet cannot find the information they need when they need it. The revolution in information technology will transform the information supply to doctors. Although most journals have in the past five years developed web versions, we are at the beginning of the revolution. The next 10 years will see unprecedented change.

Most journals will, I predict, disappear. Scientific research, most of which is funded by public money, will be made available through the world wide web. The change will come partly because researchers, particularly in the United States, resent the large profits

221

made by publishers. But more importantly it will happen because it will allow scholars worldwide to access research in all fields free from their desks. The role of journals will be less to publish research and more to find the small amount of research that matters to clinicians and present it in a way that is useful and appealing. This should reduce the pressure on doctors. The barriers to this happening are not technological but rather to do with business and culture.

The doctors' problem of not being able to find the information they need when they need it might also be solved by technology - but this will depend on technological advances. Machines will be built that will answer within a few seconds the complex questions that arise when doctors meet with patients. The machines will also guide and prompt doctors.

Epilogue

Key considerations
in
surgical publishing

M. Schein

Professor of Surgery, Cornell University Medical College
& Bronx Lebanon Hospital, New York, U.S.A.

J. R. Farndon

Professor and Head of Division, University of Bristol &
Consultant Surgeon, Bristol Royal Infirmary, Bristol, UK.

A. Fingerhut

Chief of Service, Digestive Surgery, Centre Hospitalier
Intercommunal, Poissy, France & Associate Professor of Surgery
Louisiana State University Medical School
New Orleans, LA, U.S.A.

We hope that a few of you will have enjoyed reading this book on surgical publishing. In this epilogue we would like to leave you with a few key considerations.

Considerations on why to publish [1]

Egoistic motives include the strive for academic and/or professional promotion, which, in turn, may be associated with financial gain, the will to improve one's knowledge and judgement, and the development of professional contacts. Altruistic motives are the desire to generate and disseminate knowledge.

The more you write and publish the longer is your list of publications. The more publications you have the better should be your writing ability. The better you write the greater the chance of your papers being accepted by leading journals. The more you are published in top journals the greater likelihood of your papers being cited by others. The more you are published and cited the higher your score on the impact factor and citation index lists.

While most authors will not admit that one of the strongest motives to writing is seeing their own name in print, this is the truth and nothing is wrong with it. The sum of all above is 'fame and fun' as Richard Feynman, the Nobel laureate physicist, called it 'The pleasure of finding things out'.

Considerations on what to write [2]

Don't fool yourself. Your first paper won't appear with earth-shattering findings in the *New England Journal of Medicine* or *The Lancet*. The first published paper of most giants in surgery was a case report or a limited retrospective clinical experience. Start modestly and aim higher later.

Any of your patients can be written about, especially if offering any novel aspect and if it is thoroughly researched and well written. Do not shy away from reviewing and writing about your or your department's clinical experience if you think that it can offer another perspective. Even if published 'only' in one of your regional or national journals it may be of great value to your community. Not only 'perfect results' or 'positive findings' of a study need to be published. Admire the zero mortality and morbidity rates from the ivory towers - published in the *Annals of Surgery* - but try to write up your centre's more modest experience and results. In order for you and us to improve, we need to know how are we doing in the 'real world' away from the ivory towers.

Before deciding 'what should I write' you should know 'what has been written'. Doing so, very soon you will realize that you could do it as well, or even better. Follow Faulkner's advice: 'Read, read, read everything - trash, classics, good and bad, and see how they do it. Read! You'll absorb it. Then write'. Whenever you are bothered by a dilemma for which you cannot find the 'correct' answer, think that this is something to be researched, better defined and, perhaps, written up. Don't be lazy, go to the library and search and cross-search in textbooks and journals. Always use the electronic Pubmed-Medline search machines. The condition or dilemma you are confronted with is probably more common than you thought.

Considerations on where to publish [3]

Your chief goals are the greatest readership, a prestigious, high-impact journal, speedy editorial process and a fair chance of acceptance. The potential 'market' for your manuscript is huge. It is not the end of the world if the *BJS*, for example, rejects your masterpiece. If you try hard enough each of your manuscripts will eventually be accepted by some journal.

Choose the audience (general, specialized, local?), always consult the 'instructions to authors' of the journal(s) targeted and assess objectively the value of your paper. You do not want to submit a technical paper to a theoretical journal or a banal case report to *The Lancet*. Focus on a limited list of journals, which represents a spectrum of qualities tailored to the value of your manuscripts. With time, you will learn to satisfy their editors while the latter may eventually learn to appreciate your work.

The key elements of a successful submission are to assess the value of your manuscript, to understand the publishing market, to study the target journal(s), to tailor your manuscript to the latter and, most importantly, to get learned advice from someone who is very experienced.

Considerations on the generation of an idea [4]

While ideas are plentiful, only the novice and naive think that all ideas are publishable. Only by repeatedly formulating ideas worthy of publication and bringing them to fruition will you be able to shade off your publishing naivety. It was Ernest Hemingway who said: 'The most essential gift for a good writer is a built-in, shockproof, shit detector. This is the writers' radar and all great writers have had it'.

A review article has to 'close a gap' that has not been well covered in recent major texts and journals. Ask yourself: is the topic of enough interest to capture the reader and the reviewers? Is it controversial enough to allow a stimulating discussion? Review articles, as original studies, can be tailored to the various journals. Leading journals may accept a review by the world's expert on the laparoscopic management of pancreatic carcinoma. There are, however, low-key journals that may publish your educational review on postoperative fever. Beware of claiming the 'first reported case of...'. What you think has been never published may be rare, what you suggest is rare may actually be quite common, provided that you search the literature thoroughly.

The operative technique you wish to describe has to be novel, offering a new solution to an old or new problem. Resist the temptation to perform a surgical gimmick only for the sake of its publication (e.g. laparoscopic resection of sebaceous cyst). As Sholem Asch said: 'Writing comes more easy if you have something to say'.

Not only surgical giants and 'known authorities' in their field have the right to express their opinions. If you have something valuable to say, say it clearly. It might not be accepted as an editorial or a leading article, but as a 'letter to the editor' it has a fair chance. In fact, a well edited correspondence section is one of the most well read parts of any journal.

Considerations on getting started [5]

Before you start, have a general idea of what you want to say. Preparing an outline may help. Simmer the outline for a while but do not overcook it for there may be others out there with a similar idea and plan. At this stage the results of the study must be ready. Check and recheck all numbers and figures, avoiding any embarrassing discrepancies and errors.

Tame the relevant literature by whatever means. Highlight or underline the points you wish to use, and then organize them in tables or piles. A large desk or floor is useful. Get the full text version of the papers you plan to use in your bibliography. Citing only Medline abstracts is easier but it means that you cheat yourself and the readers. According to Arthur Baue: 'Citation of secondary sources results in continued myths, misquotations, and incorrect citations. It is frustrating to seek a reference that is incorrectly cited. It is fun however, to track down and read the primary source'.

Instead of sitting in front of a blank sheet or screen take a walk, think and talk to yourself. Then try again. Writing is tough for all of us. Even Molière said: 'I always do the first line well, but I have trouble doing the others'.

Considerations on writing the manuscript [6]

The materials and methods (what you did) and results (what you found) are the body of your manuscript; start with them. Only then add the skeleton - introduction (why you wrote this paper) - and the heart - discussion (what you feel about it). The abstract comes last, as stated by Pascal Pennées: 'The last thing one settles in writing ... is what one should put in first'. The abstract alone should convey to the reader all that you did and found, and what it means. If published, most readers will never see the full version of your paper but only the electronic version of your abstract. 'There is no better writing exercise than composing an abstract' (Arthur Baue). Avoid any discrepancies between the abstract and the body of the paper because it irritates the reviewers and biases the validity of the report.

Your manuscript should be 'self-contained'. A statement such as 'the methods were described previously' might enrage the reviewers and frustrate the readers. Avoid duplications and redundancies; say what you have to say once only. Do not disclose results in the introduction, do not shift portions of the materials and methods into the results, do not repeat results in the discussion, do not introduce results or other studies in the discussion, and do not repeat data shown in the text in the tables.

Do not be biased in selecting literature for your bibliography. Be aware that the reviewers of your manuscript are experts in their field; they know the relevant literature and may 'search' it on their computers, immediately revealing your omissions. Never, we repeat, never cite a reference without reading it entirely for it is misleading and an intellectual crime. US authors tend to cite US papers and British authors tend to cite British papers. You do not want to be narrow minded in the global era: cite any study that is appropriate.

Be original. Do not plagiarize; always use your own language. It is easier to 'copy and paste' entire paragraphs from the Medline but you do not want to do this. Your discussion has to focus on your own results and compare your findings with those of others. It should not be an exhaustive review of the literature if it is not a review article. Be frank; by disclosing in the discussion the deficiencies of your study you can disarm malicious reviewers.

Whenever you sit down - or stand up (à la Hemingway) - to continue with the manuscript, reread it from the beginning. Anthony Trollope stated: 'By reading what he has last written, just before he recommences his task, the writer can catch the tone and spirit of what he is then saying...'.

Surgical publishing may deal with boring material but must not be in itself boring. Take Voltaire's advice and be brief: 'The secret of being a bore is to tell everything'. Use simple language and try to be true rather than bombastic.

Considerations on the foreign author [7]

The assumption or 'excuse' that your paper was rejected because English is not your mother language, or because you are a foreigner, is a self-serving nonsense. Reviewers are keen and able to recognize a valuable contribution even if written in broken English. Editors will do all they can to improve your article, if they consider it publishable. If you are able to complete a reasonable manuscript in your own language, why should it not be possible to do so in English? If you are versed with the basics of scientific writing in your own language, doing so in English will be much easier as it is the novelty of your idea, the quality of your study and the organization of your manuscript that really matters, more than your mother language.

Publish also in the 'local' journals of your country. Even if Matthew said that 'a prophet is not without honour, save in his own country', being famous internationally and poorly known locally negates the purpose of your writing. Beware of professional non-medical translators who 'translate' the meaning of your thoughts into beautifully sounding English gibberish. The 'importance' of publishing varies of course between different countries. 'In America only a successful writer is important, in France all writers are important. In England no writer is important. In Australia you have to explain what a writer is' (Geoffrey Cotterell).

Considerations on the final product [8]

A surgical paper, like yummy pasta, should be well prepared but *al dente*. When overboiled it is boring to the taste buds as well as to the reader. Read and reread your final manuscript. Put it aside for a few days, read it again, then reread it aloud. As Fran Lebowitz wrote: 'In conversation you can use timing, a look, inflection, pauses. But on the page all you have is commas, dashes, the amount of syllables in a word. When I write I read everything out loud to get the right rhythm'.

Choose the title carefully; let it reflect the essence of your paper while being catchy but not too gimmicky. Walker Percy said that 'a good title should be like a good metaphor; it should intrigue without being too baffling or too obvious'. Arthur Baue suggested that 'the title is the message, not the medium'. However, according to Hemingway: 'Getting a title is a lot like drawing cards in a poker game'. 'If the title is a rhetorical question, the answer is always no. If the answer was yes, the authors would have stated it accordingly' (Arthur Baue).

How lovely it feels to seal the envelope over your finished manuscript. Be optimistic but not too hopeful. According to J. B. Priestley: 'Most writers enjoy two periods of happiness - when a glorious idea comes to mind and secondly, when a last page has been written and you haven't had time to know how much better it ought to be'.

Considerations on what an editor wants or expects from authors [9]

The reviewers and editors would like your manuscript to be perfect but this is seldom the case. The farther your manuscript is from the ideal, the more irritating it is to the reviewers, and the more likely it is to land in the garbage bin. Having had your manuscript battered by the reviewers, your last hope is that the editors will detect its virtue. Editors, however, have to read numerous manuscripts. 'That is why the message of a manuscript must be clear and up front. A subtle message will be lost, as it probably should be' (Arthur Baue).

Reviewers are busy people; your manuscript must not exasperate them. Be sure to follow the instructions to authors particular to the journal to which the manuscript is sent. See that your manuscript is clearly printed and copied. Start each section on a new page, and use paragraphs and subheadings. Sloppy presentation correlates often with sloppy contents. The editorial process is lengthy. Be patient. Wait at least 3 months before calling the editorial office; only masochists call for bad news.

Considerations on politics in surgical publishing [10]

Decide about the list of authors before conducting and writing up the study. Doing it at the end causes trouble. The number of authors should correlate with the magnitude of the manuscript; for a review article or a case report to have more than three authors is ridiculous. The three most 'prestigious spots' on any list of authors are the first, second and last. Divide them between the three people who contributed to the paper most. The 'lonely author syndrome' of a large clinical study means that the author failed to acknowledge colleagues who deserve coauthorship.

Do not provide your colleagues with 'gift authorship' which, as free lunches, are rarely appreciated. They would add it to their curricula vitae without even bothering to read it. Do not accept authorship from others without having contributed significantly to the paper. Remember that your reputation is more important than your list of publications. 'You can fire your secretary, divorce your spouse, abandon your children. But they remain your coauthors forever' (Ellen Goodman).

231

Considerations of the editorial desk [11]

Contrary to what you may believe, manuscripts submitted by members of the editorial board of a journal are scrutinized as severely as yours. Their only advantage is that they know better how reviewers and editors think and what they want. You will know it as well by reading this entire book.

We agree. Editors and reviewers are a pain in the ... but, nevertheless, without them our world of scholarship would be chaotic and meaningless. But go on, bash at your critics, most writers do. 'Nature fits all her children with something to do; he who would write and can't write, can surely review' (James Russell Powell).

Considerations on the rejected article [12]

Do you wish to know what the reviewers who rejected your paper are like? Look at your local academic leaders and professors: bright, talented, honest but occasionally prejudiced, biased and even dogmatic. Do not waste energy on anger and self-pity but promptly revise and resubmit your manuscript based on the reviewers' comments with which you do agree. 'Listen carefully to first criticisms of your work. Note just what it is about your work that the critics don't like - then cultivate it, that's the part ... that's individual and worth keeping' (Jean Cocteau).

Do not despair. Somewhere along the line, perhaps even at the third or fifth journal, there will be someone who understands your idea and message. For 'in literature, as in love, we are astonished at what is chosen by others' (Andre Maurois). When rejected, do not argue with the publishers. That you are right and they are wrong won't help. Do not imitate Henry James who, when asked to delete a few words from a 5000-word article, said: 'I have performed the necessary butchery. Here is the bleeding corpse'.

Do not park the rejected manuscript at your driveway to accumulate rust. Trade it in as soon as possible and as many times as required.

Considerations on ethics of writing [13]

Even the best salami loses flavour at its cut edges. The more it is sliced into tiny pieces, the more of its original taste you lose. Likewise, do not slice your study into tasteless thin pieces. Fish tastes best when fresh out of the water. A day later, at brunch, its bitterness has to be disguised with mayonnaise. It is the same with your study; if reprocessed - duplicated in another journal - it will offend your colleagues and may even cause food poisoning.

Words, when shaped into sentences, paragraphs and ideas, become the intellectual property of their original author. The best antidote to plagiarism is always to cite your sources. 'If you copy from one author it's plagiarism. If you copy from two, it's research' (Wilson Mizner).

Conclusions

We hope that you will become a successful surgical writer and, sooner or later, you will do it naturally, in your own way. As Somerset Maugham said: 'There are three rules for writing ... unfortunately, no one knows what they are', and to the critics of this chapter, who surely will claim that we have used too many quotations, let us cite from Winston Churchill: 'It is a good thing for an uneducated man to read books of quotations'.

Obviously, there is nothing new in the ideas included in this book, for scientific writing is ageless. Our aim, however, was to digest the essence of publishing specifically for you, the surgeon. To paraphrase Baue [14]: we wish to offer to the young or old surgeon to put words on paper, write and rewrite, and rewrite again. Surgical literature needs all worthwhile contributions, reports and ideas.

References

1   Schein M, Farndon JR, Fingerhut A. Why should a surgeon publish? *Br J Surg* 2000; 87: 3-5.

2   O'Connell PR. What should surgeons write? *Br J Surg* 2000; 87: 132-4.

3   Schein M, Fingerhut A. Where can surgeons publish? *Br J Surg* 2000; 87: 261-4.

4   Sarr MG. Generating an idea: will it be publishable? *Br J Surg* 2000; 87: 388-9.

5   Alderson D. On getting started. *Br J Surg* 2000; 87: 532-3.

6   Wells SA. Writing the manuscript. *Br J Surg* 2000; 87: 691-2.

7   Rothmund M, Fingerhut A. The 'foreign' author. *Br J Surg* 2000; 87: 835-6.

8   Murie JA. The final product. *Br J Surg* 2000; 87: 980-2.

9   Organ CH. What an editor wants or expects from authors. *Br J Surg* 2000; 87: 1123-4.

10   Laitman CJ, Rikkers LF. Politics in surgical publishing. *Br J Surg* 2000; 87: 1284-6.

11   Farndon JR, Murie JA. On the editor's desk. *Br J Surg* 2000; 87: 1444-7.

12   Guillou PJ, Earnshaw JJ. Dealing with the rejected article. *Br J Surg* 2000; 87: 1603-4.

13   Farthing MJG. Research misconduct: diagnosis, treatment and prevention. *Br J Surg* 2000; 87: 1605-9.

14   Baue A. Reflections of a former editor. *Arch Surg.* 1993; 128: 1305-14.

Appendix I

Guidelines
on good
publication practice

Committee on Publication Ethics (COPE)
Reproduced with the kind permission
of
the BMJ Publishing Group
from
The COPE Report 1999.

Why the guidelines were developed

COPE was founded in 1997 to address breaches of research and publication ethics. A voluntary body providing a discussion forum and advice for scientific editors, it aims to find practical ways of dealing with the issues, and to develop good practice.

We thought it essential to attempt to define best practice in the ethics of scientific publishing. These guidelines should be useful for authors, editors, editorial board members, readers, owners of journals, and publishers.

Intellectual honesty should be actively encouraged in all medical and scientific courses of study, and used to inform publication ethics and prevent misconduct. It is with that in mind that these guidelines have been produced.

Details of other guidelines on the ethics of research and published codes of conduct are listed in the *Appendix*.

How the guidelines were developed

The guidelines were developed from a preliminary version drafted by individual members of the committee, which was then submitted to extensive consultation. They address: study design and ethical approval, data analysis, authorship, conflict of interests, the peer review process, redundant publication, plagiarism, duties of editors, media relations, advertising, and how to deal with misconduct.

What they aim to do

These guidelines are intended to be advisory rather than prescriptive, and to evolve over time. We hope that they will be disseminated widely, endorsed by editors, and refined by those who use them.

1   Study design and ethical approval

2   Data analysis

3   Authorship

4   Conflicts of interest

5   Peer review

6   Redundant publication

7   Plagiarism

8   Duties of editors

9   Media relations

10   Advertising

Dealing with misconduct

Appendix

Acknowledgement

The following are gratefully acknowledged for their contribution to the drafting of these guidelines:

Philip Fulford (Coordinator)

Professor Michael Doherty

Ms Jane Smith

Dr Richard Smith

Dr Fiona Godlee

Dr Peter Wilmshurst

Dr Richard Horton

Professor Michael Farthing

Other members of COPE

Delegates to the Meeting on April 27 1999

Other corresponding editors

1   Study design and ethical approval

Definition

Good research should be well justified, well planned, appropriately designed, and ethically approved. To conduct research to a lower standard may constitute misconduct.

Action

1. Laboratory and clinical research should be driven by protocol; pilot studies should have a written rationale.
2. Research protocols should seek to answer specific questions, rather than just collect data.
3. Protocols must be carefully agreed by all contributors and collaborators, including, if appropriate, the participants.
4. The final protocol should form part of the research record.
5. Early agreement on the precise roles of the contributors and collaborators, and on matters of authorship and publication, is advised.
6. Statistical issues should be considered early in study design, including power calculations, to ensure there are neither too few nor too many participants.
7. Formal and documented ethical approval from an appropriately constituted research ethics committee is required for all studies involving people, medical records, and anonymised human tissues.
8. Use of human tissues in research should conform to the highest ethical standards, such as those recommended by the Nuffield Council on Bioethics.
9. Fully informed consent should always be sought. It may not always be possible, however, and in such circumstances, an appropriately constituted research ethics committee should decide if this is ethically acceptable.

10. When participants are unable to give fully informed consent, research should follow international guidelines, such as those of the Council for International Organizations of Medical Sciences (CIOMS).

11. Animal experiments require full compliance with local, national, ethical, and regulatory principles, and local licensing arrangements. International standards vary.

12. Formal supervision, usually the responsibility of the principal investigator, should be provided for all research projects: this must include quality control, and the frequent review and long term retention (may be up to 15 years) of all records and primary outputs.

2   Data analysis

Definition

Data should be appropriately analysed, but inappropriate analysis does not necessarily amount to misconduct. Fabrication and falsification of data do constitute misconduct.

Action

1. All sources and methods used to obtain and analyse data, including any electronic pre-processing, should be fully disclosed; detailed explanations should be provided for any exclusions.

2. Methods of analysis must be explained in detail, and referenced, if they are not in common use.

3. The post hoc analysis of subgroups is acceptable, as long as this is disclosed. Failure to disclose that the analysis was post hoc is unacceptable.

4. The discussion section of a paper should mention any issues of bias which have been considered, and explain how they have been dealt with in the design and interpretation of the study.

3   Authorship

Definition

There is no universally agreed definition of authorship, although attempts have been made (*see Appendix to these guidelines*). As a minimum, authors should take responsibility for a particular section of the study.

Action

1.   The award of authorship should balance intellectual contributions to the conception, design, analysis and writing of the study against the collection of data and other routine work. If there is no task that can reasonably be attributed to a particular individual, then that individual should not be credited with authorship.
2.   To avoid disputes over attribution of academic credit, it is helpful to decide early on in the planning of a research project who will be credited as authors, as contributors, and who will be acknowledged.
3.   All authors must take public responsibility for the content of their paper. The multidisciplinary nature of much research can make this difficult, but this can be resolved by the disclosure of individual contributions.
4.   Careful reading of the target journal's 'Advice to Authors' is advised, in the light of current uncertainties.

4   Conflicts of interest

Definition

Conflicts of interest comprise those which may not be fully apparent and which may influence the judgment of author, reviewers, and editors.

They have been described as those which, when revealed later, would make a reasonable reader feel misled or deceived.

They may be personal, commercial, political, academic or financial.

'Financial' interests may include employment, research funding, stock or share ownership, payment for lectures or travel, consultancies and company support for staff.

Action

1. Such interests, where relevant, must be declared to editors by researchers, authors, and reviewers.
2. Editors should also disclose relevant conflicts of interest to their readers. If in doubt, disclose. Sometimes editors may need to withdraw from the review and selection process for the relevant submission.

5   Peer review

Definition

Peer reviewers are external experts chosen by editors to provide written opinions, with the aim of improving the study.

Working methods vary from journal to journal, but some use open procedures in which the name of the reviewer is disclosed, together with the full or 'edited' report.

Action

1. Suggestions from authors as to who might act as reviewers are often useful, but there should be no obligation on editors to use those suggested.

2. The duty of confidentiality in the assessment of a manuscript must be maintained by expert reviewers, and this extends to reviewers' colleagues who may be asked (with the editor's permission) to give opinions on specific sections.
3. The submitted manuscript should not be retained or copied.
4. Reviewers and editors should not make any use of the data, arguments, or interpretations, unless they have the authors' permission.
5. Reviewers should provide speedy, accurate, courteous, unbiased and justifiable reports.
6. If reviewers suspect misconduct, they should write in confidence to the editor.
7. Journals should publish accurate descriptions of their peer review, selection, and appeals processes.
8. Journals should also provide regular audits of their acceptance rates and publication times.

6 Redundant publication

Definition

Redundant publication occurs when two or more papers, without full cross reference, share the same hypothesis, data, discussion points, or conclusions.

Action

1. Published studies do not need to be repeated unless further confirmation is required.
2. Previous publication of an abstract during the proceedings of meetings does not preclude subsequent submission for publication, but full disclosure should be made at the time of submission.
3. Re-publication of a paper in another language is acceptable, provided that there is full and prominent disclosure of its original source at the time of submission.

4. At the time of submission, authors should disclose details of related papers, even if in a different language, and similar papers in press.

7   Plagiarism

Definition

Plagiarism ranges from the unreferenced use of others' published and unpublished ideas, including research grant applications to submission under 'new' authorship of a complete paper, sometimes in a different language.

It may occur at any stage of planning, research, writing, or publication: it applies to print and electronic versions.

Action

1. All sources should be disclosed, and if large amounts of other people's written or illustrative material is to be used, permission must be sought.

8   Duties of editors

Definition

Editors are the stewards of journals. They usually take over their journal from the previous editor(s) and always want to hand over the journal in good shape.

Most editors provide direction for the journal and build a strong management team.

They must consider and balance the interests of many constituents, including readers, authors, staff, owners, editorial board members, advertisers and the media.

Action

1. Editors' decisions to accept or reject a paper for publication should be based only on the paper's importance, originality, and clarity, and the study's relevance to the remit of the journal.
2. Studies that challenge previous work published in the journal should be given an especially sympathetic hearing.
3. Studies reporting negative results should not be excluded.
4. All original studies should be peer reviewed before publication, taking into full account possible bias due to related or conflicting interests.
5. Editors must treat all submitted papers as confidential.
6. When a published paper is subsequently found to contain major flaws, editors must accept responsibility for correcting the record prominently and promptly.

9 Media relations

Definition

Medical research findings are of increasing interest to the print and broadcast media.

Journalists may attend scientific meetings at which preliminary research findings are presented, leading to their premature publication in the mass media.

Action

1. Authors approached by the media should give as balanced an account of their work as possible, ensuring that they point out where evidence ends and speculation begins.
2. Simultaneous publication in the mass media and a peer reviewed journal is advised, as this usually means that enough evidence and data have been provided to satisfy informed and critical readers.

3. Where this is not possible, authors should help journalists to produce accurate reports, but refrain from supplying additional data.

4. All efforts should be made to ensure that patients who have helped with the research should be informed of the results by the authors before the mass media, especially if there are clinical implications.

5. Authors should be advised by the organisers if journalists are to attend scientific meetings.

6. It may be helpful to authors to be advised of any media policies operated by the journal in which their work is to be published.

10   Advertising

Definition

Many scientific journals and meetings derive significant income from advertising.

Reprints may also be lucrative.

Action

1. Editorial decisions must not be influenced by advertising revenue or reprint potential: editorial and advertising administration must be clearly separated.

2. Advertisements that mislead must be refused, and editors must be willing to publish criticisms, according to the same criteria used for material in the rest of the journal.

3. Reprints should be published as they appear in the journal unless a correction is to be added.

Dealing with misconduct

1   Principles

1. The general principle confirming misconduct is intention to cause others to regard as true that which is not true.
2. The examination of misconduct must therefore focus, not only on the particular act or omission, but also on the intention of the researcher, author, editor, reviewer or publisher involved.
3. Deception may be by intention, by reckless disregard of possible consequences, or by negligence. It is implicit, therefore, that 'best practice' requires complete honesty, with full disclosure.
4. Codes of practice may raise awareness, but can never be exhaustive.

2   Investigating misconduct

1. Editors should not simply reject papers that raise questions of misconduct. They are ethically obliged to pursue the case. However, knowing how to investigate and respond to possible cases of misconduct is difficult.
2. COPE is always willing to advise, but for legal reasons, can only advise on anonymised cases.
3. It is for the editor to decide what action to take.

3   Serious misconduct

1. Editors must take all allegations and suspicions of misconduct seriously, but they must recognise that they do not usually have either the legal legitimacy or the means to conduct investigations into serious cases.
2. The editor must decide when to alert the employers of the accused author(s).
3. Some evidence is required, but if employers have a process for investigating accusations - as they are increasingly required to do - then editors do not need to assemble a complete case. Indeed, it

may be ethically unsound for editors to do so, because such action usually means consulting experts, so spreading abroad serious questions about the author(s).

4. If editors are presented with convincing evidence - perhaps by reviewers - of serious misconduct, they should immediately pass this on to the employers, notifying the author(s) that they are doing so.

5. If accusations of serious misconduct are not accompanied by convincing evidence, then editors should confidentially seek expert advice.

6. If the experts raise serious questions about the research, then editors should notify the employers.

7. If the experts find no evidence of misconduct, the editorial processes should proceed in the normal way.

8. If presented with convincing evidence of serious misconduct, where there is no employer to whom this can be referred, and the author(s) are registered doctors, cases can be referred to the General Medical Council.

9. If, however, there is no organisation with the legitimacy and the means to conduct an investigation, then the editor may decide that the case is sufficiently important to warrant publishing something in the journal. Legal advice will then be essential.

10. If editors are convinced that an employer has not conducted an adequate investigation of a serious accusation, they may feel that publication of a notice in the journal is warranted. Legal advice will be essential.

11. Authors should be given the opportunity to respond to accusations of serious misconduct

4 *Less serious misconduct*

1. Editors may judge that it is not necessary to involve employers in less serious cases of misconduct, such as redundant publication, deception over authorship, or failure to declare conflict of interest. Sometimes the evidence may speak for itself, although it may be wise to appoint an independent expert.

2. Editors should remember that accusations of even minor misconduct may have serious implications for the author(s), and it may then be necessary to ask the employers to investigate.

3. Authors should be given the opportunity to respond to any charge of minor misconduct.

4. If convinced of wrongdoing, editors may wish to adopt some of the sanctions outlined below.

5   Sanctions

Sanctions may be applied separately or combined. The following are ranked in approximate order of severity:

1. A letter of explanation (and education) to the authors, where there appears to be a genuine misunderstanding of principles.

2. A letter of reprimand and warning as to future conduct.

3. A formal letter to the relevant head of institution or funding body.

4. Publication of a notice of redundant publication or plagiarism.

5. An editorial giving full details of the misconduct.

6. Refusal to accept future submissions from the individual, unit, or institution responsible for the misconduct, for a stated period.

7. Formal withdrawal or retraction of the paper from the scientific literature, informing other editors and the indexing authorities.

8. Reporting the case to the General Medical Council, or other such authority or organisation which can investigate and act with due process.

Appendix

The Association of the British Pharmaceutical Industry. *Facilities for non-patient volunteer studies*. London: APBI, 1989.

The Association of the British Pharmaceutical Industry. *Guidelines for medical experiments in non-patient human volunteers*. London: ABPI, 1990.

ABPI fact sheets and guidance notes:

Clinical trials and compensation guidelines, January 1991.

Guidelines for phase IV clinical trials, September 1993.

Guidelines on the conduct of investigator site audits, January 1994.

Relationship between the medical profession and the pharmaceutical industry, June 1994.

Good clinical trial practice, November 1995.

Patient information and consents for clinical trials, May 1997.

Guidelines on the structure of a formal agreement to conduct sponsored clinical research, July 1998.

Good clinical research practice, July 1998.

Council for International Organizations of Medical Sciences (CIOMS). *International Guidelines for Ethical Review of Epidemiological Studies.* Geneva: WHO, 1991.

General Medical Council. Good medical practice guidelines series:

Consent, February 1999.

Confidentiality, October 1995.

Transplantation of organs from live donors, November 1992.

International Committee of Medical Journal Editors (ICMJE). Uniform requirements for manuscripts submitted to biomedical journals. *JAMA* 1997; 277: 927-34.

Medical Research Council. *Policy and procedure for inquiring into allegations of scientific misconduct.* London: MRC, 1997.

Medical Research Council. *The ethical conduct of research on the mentally incapacitated.* London: MRC, 1991.

Medical Research Council. *The ethical conduct of research on children.* London: MRC, 1991.

Medical Research Council. *Responsibility in the use of animals in medical research.* London: MRC, 1993.

Medical Research Council. *Responsibility in the use of personal medical information for research. Principles and guidelines to practice.* London: MRC, 1985.

Medical Research Council. *MRC Guidelines for good clinical practice in clinical trials.* London: MRC, 1998.

Medical Research Council. *Principles in the assessment and conduct of medical research and publicising results.* London: MRC, 1995.

Nuffield Council on Bioethics. *Human tissue: Ethical and legal issues.* London: Nuffield Council on Bioethics, 1995.

Royal College of Physicians. *Research involving patients.* London: RCP, 1990.

Appendix II

Improving the quality of reports
of meta-analyses of
randomised controlled trials:
the QUOROM statement

The QUOROM Group

David Moher, Deborah J Cook, Susan Eastwood, Ingram
Olkin, Drummond Rennie, Donna F Stroup, for the
QUOROM Group*
*Other members listed at end of paper

Reproduced with the kind permission
of The Lancet 1999; 354: 1896-900.

University of Ottawa, Thomas C Chalmers Centre for Systematic Reviews, Ottawa (D Moher MSc); McMaster University, Hamilton (D J Cook MD), Ontario, Canada; University of California, San Francisco (S Eastwood ELS(D)); Stanford University, Stanford, CA (I Olkin PhD); JAMA, Chicago, IL (D Rennie PhD); and Centers for Disease Control and Prevention, Atlanta, GA, USA (D F Stroup PhD)

Correspondence to: Dr David Moher, Thomas C Chalmers Centre for Systematic Reviews, Children's Hospital of Eastern Ontario Research Institute, 401 Smyth Road, Ottawa, Ontario K1H 8L1, Canada (e-mail dmoher@uottawa.ca)

Summary

Background

The Quality of Reporting of Meta-analyses (QUOROM) conference was convened to address standards for improving the quality of reporting of meta-analyses of clinical randomised controlled trials (RCTs).

Methods

The QUOROM group consisted of 30 clinical epidemiologists, clinicians, statisticians, editors, and researchers. In conference, the group was asked to identify items they thought should be included in a checklist of standards. Whenever possible, checklist items were guided by research evidence suggesting that failure to adhere to the item proposed could lead to biased results. A modified Delphi technique was used in assessing candidate items.

Findings

The conference resulted in the QUOROM statement, a checklist, and a flow diagram. The checklist describes our preferred way to present the abstract, introduction, methods, results, and discussion sections of a report of a meta-analysis. It is organised into 21 headings and subheadings regarding searches, selection, validity assessment, data abstraction, study characteristics, and quantitative data synthesis, and in the results with 'trial flow', study characteristics, and quantitative data synthesis; research documentation was identified for eight of the 18 items. The flow diagram provides information about both the numbers of RCTs identified, included, and excluded and the reasons for exclusion of trials.

Interpretation

We hope this report will generate further thought about ways to improve the quality of reports of meta-analyses of RCTs and that interested readers, reviewers, researchers, and editors will use the QUOROM statement and generate ideas for its improvement.

Introduction

Health-care providers and other decision-makers now have, among their information resources, a form of clinical report called the meta-analysis,[1-4] a review in which bias has been reduced by the systematic identification, appraisal, synthesis, and, if relevant, statistical aggregation of all relevant studies on a specific topic according to a predetermined and explicit method.[3] The number of published meta-analyses has increased substantially in the past decade.[5] These integrative articles can be helpful for clinical decisions, and they may also serve as the policy foundation for evidence-based practice guidelines, economic evaluations, and future research agendas. The value of meta-analysis is evident in the work of the international Cochrane Collaboration,[6,7] the primary purpose of which is to generate and disseminate high-quality systematic reviews of health-care interventions.

Like any research enterprise, particularly one that is observational, the meta-analysis of evidence can be flawed. Accordingly, the process by which meta-analyses are carried out has undergone scrutiny. A 1987 survey of 86 English-language meta-analyses[8] assessed each publication on 23 items from six content areas judged important in the conduct and reporting of a meta-analysis of randomised trials: study design, combinability, control of bias, statistical analysis, sensitivity analysis, and problems of applicability. The survey results showed that only 24 (28%) of the 86 meta-analyses reported that all six content areas had been addressed. The updated survey, which included more recently published meta-analyses, showed little improvement in the rigour with which they were reported.[9]

Several publications have described the science of reviewing research,[1] differences among narrative reviews, systematic reviews, and meta-analyses,[2] and how to carry out,[3,4,10] critically appraise,[11-15] and apply[16] meta-analyses in practice. The increase in the number of meta-analyses published has highlighted such issues as discordant meta-analyses on the same topic[17] and discordant meta-analyses and randomised-trial results on the same question.[18]

An important consideration in interpretation and use of meta-analyses is to ascertain that the investigators who did the meta-analysis not only report explicitly the methods they used to analyse the articles they reviewed, but also report the methods used in the research articles they analysed. The meta-analytical review methods used may not be provided when a paper is initially submitted: even when they are, other factors such as page limitations, peer review, and editorial decisions may change the content and format of the report before publication.

Several investigators have suggested guidelines for reporting of meta-analyses.[3,19] However, a consensus across disciplines has not developed. After the initiative to improve the quality of reporting of randomised controlled trials (RCTs),[20-22] we organised the Quality of Reporting of Meta-analyses (QUOROM) conference to address these issues as they relate to meta-analyses of RCTs. This report summarises the proceedings of that conference. The issues discussed might also be useful for reporting of systematic reviews (i.e. meta-analysis, as defined above, without statistical aggregation), particularly of RCTs.

Methods

The QUOROM steering committee began with a comprehensive review of publications on the conduct and reporting of meta-analyses. The databases searched included MEDLINE and the Cochrane Library,[23] which consists of the Cochrane Database of Systematic Reviews, the Cochrane Controlled Trials Register, the York Database of Abstracts of Reviews of Effectiveness, and the Cochrane Review Methodology Database. We examined reference lists of the retrieved articles and individual personal files. Articles of potential relevance were retrieved and critically appraised by the QUOROM steering committee. The committee generated a draft agenda for the conference, which included six domains requiring discussion and debate. The content areas were slightly modified during preliminary discussions at the conference and are reported as: the search for the evidence; decision-making on which evidence to include; description of the characteristics of primary studies; quantitative data synthesis; reliability and issues related to internal validity (or quality); and clinical implications related to external validity (or generalisability).

In planning the QUOROM conference, the steering committee identified clinical epidemiologists, clinicians, statisticians, and researchers who conduct meta-analysis as well as editors from the UK and North America who are interested in meta-analysis. These 30 individuals were invited to a conference in Chicago on Oct 2-3, 1996. Participants were surveyed before the meeting to elicit their views on current reporting standards of meta-analyses and whether these needed improvement. In addition, they were sent relevant citations for review and were asked to indicate in which of the six groups they wished to participate.

The conference included small-group and plenary sessions. Each small group had a facilitator who was a member of the steering committee and was responsible for ensuring the discussions of as many as possible of the issues relevant to their specific remit. Each small group also had a recorder, who was responsible for documenting

Improving the quality of reports of meta-analyses of randomised controlled trials: the QUOROM statement checklist

Heading	Subheading	Descriptor	Reported? (Y/N)	Page number
Title		Identify the report as a meta-analysis (or systematic review) of RCTs[26]		
Abstract		**Describe**		
	Objectives	The clinical question explicitly		
	Data sources	The databases (i.e. list) and other information sources		
	Review methods	The selection criteria (i.e. population, intervention, outcome, and study design); methods for validity assessment, data abstraction, and study characteristics, and quantitative data synthesis in sufficient detail to permit replication		
	Results	Characteristics of the RCTs included and excluded; qualitative and quantitative findings (i.e. point estimates and confidence intervals); and subgroup analyses		
	Conclusion	The main results		
Introduction		**Describe**		
		The explicit clinical problem, biological rationale for the intervention, and rationale for review		
Methods	Searching	The information sources, in detail[28] (e.g. databases, registers, personal files, expert informants, agencies, hand-searching), and any restrictions (years considered, publication status,[29] language of publication[30,31])		
	Selection	The inclusion and exclusion criteria (defining population, intervention, principal outcomes, and study design[32]		

Heading	Subheading	Descriptor	Reported? (Y/N)	Page number
Methods contd:-	Validity assessment	The criteria and process used (e.g. masked conditions, quality assessment and their findings[33-36]		
	Data abstraction	The process or processes used (e.g. completed independently, in duplicate)[35,36]		
	Study characteristics	The type of study design, participants' characteristics, details of intervention, outcome definitions, &c.,[37] and how clincal heterogeneity was assessed		
	Quantitative data synthesis	The principal measures of effect (e.g. relative risk), method of combining results (statistical testing and confidence intervals), handling of missing data; how statistical heterogeneity was assessed;[38] a rationale for any a-priori sensitivity and subgroup analyses; and any assessment of publication bias[39]		
Results	Trial flow	Provide a meta-analysis profile summarising trial flow (see figure)		
	Study characteristics	Present descriptive data for each trial (e.g. age, sample size, intervention, dose duration, follow-up period)		
	Quantitative data synthesis	Report agreement on the selection and validity assessment; present simple summary results (for each treatment group in each trial, for each primary outcome); present data needed to calculate effect sizes and confidence intervals in intention-to-treat analyses (e.g. 2x2 tables of counts, means and SDs, proportions)		
Discussion		Summarise key findings; discuss clinical inferences based on internal and external validity; interpret the results in light of the totality of available evidence; describe potential biases in the review process (e.g. publication bias); and suggest a future research agenda		

the main points and the consensus on each issue discussed during that session; the recorder presented the group's consensus during the plenary sessions. During the plenary sessions, an elected scribe from each small group was responsible for recording the principal points relevant to that group's charge that arose during the plenary discussion.

The participants in each small group were asked to identify items that they thought should be included in a checklist of standards that would be useful for investigators, editors, and peer reviewers. We asked that, whenever possible, items included in the checklist be guided by research evidence that suggested that a failure to adhere to the particular checklist item proposed could lead to biased results. For example, a substantial lack of sensitivity and specificity of MEDLINE searches is evident.[24] Therefore, the checklist suggests that investigators explicitly describe all search strategies used to locate articles for inclusion in a meta-analysis. In considering whether candidate items were essential, each subgroup used a modified Delphi technique[25] that was replicated in the plenary sessions.

Results

The conference resulted in the QUOROM statement: a checklist (table) and a flow diagram (figure). The checklist of standards for reporting of meta-analyses describes our preferred way to present the abstract, introduction, methods, results, and discussion sections of a report of a meta-analysis. The checklist is organised into 21 headings and subheadings to encourage authors to provide readers with information on searches, selection, validity assessment, data abstraction, study characteristics, quantitative data synthesis, and trial flow. Authors are asked to provide a flow diagram (figure) providing information about the number of RCTs identified, included, and excluded and the reasons for excluding them.[10]

Pretesting

After development of the checklist and flow diagram, two members of the steering committee (DM, DJC) undertook pretesting with epidemiology graduate students studying meta-analysis, residents in general internal medicine, participants at a Canadian Cochrane Center workshop, and faculty members of departments of medicine and of epidemiology and biostatistics. One group of candidates for a

Improving the quality of reports of meta-analyses of randomised controlled trials: the QUOROM statement flow diagram

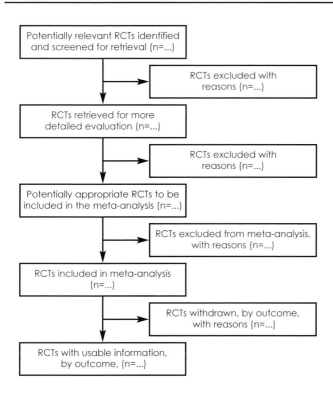

master's degree in epidemiology used the checklist and flow diagram to report their meta-analyses as if their work were being submitted for publication. Feedback from these four groups was positive, most users stating that the checklist and flow diagram would be likely to improve reporting standards. Modifications of the checklist (e.g. inclusion of a statement about major findings) and changes to the flow diagram (e.g. more detail) were incorporated.

Discussion

In developing the checklist, we identified supporting scientific evidence for only eight of 18 items to guide the reporting of meta-analyses of RCTs.[26-39] Some of this evidence is indirect. For example, we ask authors to use a structured abstract format. The supporting evidence for this item was collected by examining abstracts of original reports of individual studies[27] and may not pertain specifically to the reporting of meta-analyses. However, the QUOROM group judged this a reasonable approach by analogy with other types of research reports and pending further evidence about the merits of structured abstracts for meta-analyses.

We have asked authors to be explicit in reporting the criteria used when assessing the 'quality' of trials included in meta-analyses and the outcome of the quality assessment. There is direct and compelling evidence to support recommendations about reporting on the quality of RCTs included in a meta-analysis. A meta-analytic database of 255 obstetric RCTs provided evidence that trials with inadequate reporting of allocation concealment (i.e. keeping the intervention assignments hidden from all participants in the trial until the point of allocation) overestimated the intervention effect by 30% compared with trials in which this information was adequately reported.[33] Similar results for several disease categories and methods of quality assessment have been reported.[34] These findings suggest that inclusion of reports of low-quality RCTs in meta-analyses is likely to alter the summary measures of the intervention effect.

We also ask authors to be explicit in reporting assessment of publication bias, and we recommend that the discussion should include comments about whether the results obtained may have been influenced by such bias. Publication bias derives from the selective publishing of studies with statistically significant or directionally positive results,[40-42] and it can lead to inflated estimates of efficacy in meta-analyses. For example, trials of single alkylating agents versus multiple-agent cytotoxic chemotherapy in the treatment of ovarian cancer have been analysed.[39] Published trials yielded significant results in favour of the multiple-agent therapy, but that finding was not supported when the results of all trials - both those published and those registered but not published - were analysed.

The statement asks authors to be explicit about the publication status of reports included in a meta-analysis. Only about a third of published meta-analyses report the inclusion of unpublished data.[29,43] Although one study found that there were no substantial differences in the dimensions of study quality between published and unpublished clinical research,[42] another suggested that intervention effects reported in journals were 33% greater than those reported in doctoral dissertations.[44] The role of the 'grey literature' (difficult to locate or retrieve) was examined in 39 meta-analyses that included 467 RCTs, 102 of which were grey literature.[29] Meta-analyses limited to published trials, compared with those that included both published and grey literature, overestimated the treatment effect by an average of 12%. There is still debate between editors and investigators about the importance of including unpublished data in a meta-analysis.[43]

We have asked authors to be explicit in reporting whether they have used any restrictions on language of publication. Roughly a third of published meta-analyses have some language restrictions as part of the eligibility criteria for including individual trials.[30] The reason for such restrictions is not clear, since there is no evidence to support differences in study quality, and there is evidence that language restrictions may result in a biased summary. The reports of 127 RCTs written in English, compared with those reported in four other languages, showed little or no difference in several important methodological features.[45] Similar results have been reported elsewhere.[31] The role of language restrictions has been studied in 211 RCTs included in 18 meta-analyses in which trials published in languages other than English were included in the quantitative summary.[30] Language-restricted meta-analyses overestimated the treatment effect by only 2% on average compared with language-inclusive meta-analyses. However, the language-inclusive meta-analyses were more precise.[30]

Reports of RCTs with statistically positive results are more likely than those with negative results to be published in English.[31] Likewise, there is emerging evidence to suggest that reports of RCTs from certain countries mostly have statistically positive results.[46]

We used several methods to generate the checklist and flow diagram: a systematic review of the reporting of meta-analyses; focus groups of the steering committee; and a modified Delphi approach during the conference. Although we did not involve certain users of meta-analyses (policy-makers or patients), we formally pretested this document with representatives of several constituencies who would use the recommendations and made modifications accordingly.

The QUOROM group also discussed the format of a meta-analysis report, how best to assess the impact of the QUOROM statement, and how best to disseminate it. The format we recommend includes 15 subheadings that reflect the sequential stages in the conduct of the meta-analysis within the text of the report of a meta-analysis. The checklist included in the statement can also be used during the planning, performing, and reporting of a meta-analysis and during peer review of the report after its submission to a journal.

We delayed publication of the QUOROM statement until its impact on the editorial process had been assessed. We organised an RCT involving eight medical journals to assess the impact of use of QUOROM criteria on journal peer review. Accrual is now complete and we will report the trial results elsewhere.

After about 5 weeks of electronic posting we had received five comments from investigators, whom we thank for their thoughtful consideration of the statement. Several issues, in particular in relation to terminology, cannot be addressed in the statement at present. The QUOROM group is agreed on the importance of making changes to the checklist in the light of documented evidence and must resist changes based on opinion or anecdotal evidence unless there is a compelling rationale for doing otherwise. Nonetheless, the issues raised have been noted for consideration and discussion in future.

Several queries addressed the distinction between the meta-analysis and systematic review. As we indicate in the introduction, and throughout the statement, the QUOROM group agreed to observe the distinction as defined by the Potsdam consultation on meta-analysis.[3]

We were also asked to clarify the checklist item asking investigators to interpret their results in light of the totality of evidence. Increasingly, several meta-analyses on the same topic are reported.[47-49] If other similar reports are available, authors should discuss their results as they relate to such evidence.

For the QUOROM statement to continue to be useful, it must remain evidence based and up to date. Members of the QUOROM group need to survey the literature continually to help inform themselves about emerging evidence on reporting of meta-analyses. This information needs to be collated and presented annually for two purposes. The first is decisions on which checklist items to keep, delete, or add; these decisions can be made similarly to the selection of the original items. The second purpose is so that an up to date summary on the reporting of meta-analyses can be prepared. These efforts are being coordinated through a website. This approach is similar to the CONSORT initiative.

In summary, our choice of items to include in a meta-analysis report was based on evidence whenever possible, which implies the need to include items that can systematically influence estimates of treatment effects. Currently, we lack a detailed understanding of all the factors leading to bias in the result of a meta-analysis. Clearly, research is required to help improve the quality of reporting of meta-analyses. Such evidence may also act as a catalyst for improving the methods by which meta-analyses are conducted.

The QUOROM checklist and flow diagram are available on *The Lancet's* website [www.thelancet.com]. We hope that this document will generate further interest in the field of meta-analysis and that, like the CONSORT initiative, the QUOROM statement will become available in different languages and locations as it is disseminated. We invite interested readers, reviewers, researchers, and editors to use the QUOROM statement and generate ideas for improvement.

Contributors

David Moher, Deborah Cook, Susan Eastwood, Ingram Olkin, Drummond Rennie, and Donna Stroup developed the QUOROM statement. They all planned the meeting, participated in regular conference calls, identified and secured funding, identified and invited participants, and planned the meeting agenda. All of them helped write the report, including revisions.

QUOROM participants

D G Altman (ICRF/NHS Centre for Statistics in Medicine, Oxford, UK); J A Berlin (University of Pennsylvania, Philadelphia, PA, USA); L Bero (University of California, San Francisco, CA, USA); W DuMouchel (AT&T Laboratories, New York, NY, USA); K Dickersin (Brown University, Providence, RI, USA); J J Deeks (ICRF/NHS Centre for Statistics in Medicine, Oxford, UK); P Fontanarosa (*JAMA*, Chicago, IL, USA); N Geller (National Heart, Lung, and Blood Institute, Bethesda, MD, USA); F Godlee (*BMJ*, London, UK); S Goodman (*Annals of Internal Medicine*, Philadelphia, PA, USA); R Horton (*The Lancet*, (London, UK); P Huston (University of Ottawa,

Ottawa, Canada); A R Jadad (McMaster University, Hamilton, Canada); K Kafadar (University of Colorado, Denver, CO, USA); T Klassen (University of Alberta, Edmonton, Canada); S Morton (RAND, Santa Monica, CA, USA); C Mulrow (University of Texas, San Antonio, TX, USA); S Pyke (GlaxoWellcome, London, UK); H S Sacks (Mount Sinai School of Medicine, New York, NY, USA); K F Schulz, (Family Health International, Research Triangle Park, NC, USA); S G Thompson (Imperial College School of Medicine, London, UK); M Winker (*JAMA*, Chicago, IL, USA); S Yusuf (McMaster University, Hamilton, Canada).

Acknowledgments

We thank Iain Chalmers, Ted Colton, Sander Greenland, Brian Haynes, Edward J Huth, Alessandro Liberati, Tom Louis, Roy Pitkin, David Sackett, Trevor Sheldon, and Chris Silagy, for reviewing earlier drafts of this paper, and Jacqueline Page for helping with revisions. Financial support was provided by Abbott Laboratories, Agency for Health Care Policy & Research, GlaxoWellcome, and Merck & Co.

References

1   Mulrow CD. The medical review article: state of the science. *Ann Intern Med* 1987; 106: 485-88.
2   Cook DJ, Mulrow C, Haynes RB. Systematic reviews: synthesis of best evidence for clinical decisions. *Ann Intern Med* 1997; 126: 376-80.
3   Cook DJ, Sackett DL, Spitzer W. Methodologic guidelines for systematic reviews of randomized controlled trials in health care from the Potsdam consultation on meta-analysis. *J Clin Epidemiol* 1995; 48: 167-71.
4   Deeks J, Glanville J, Sheldon T. Undertaking systematic reviews of research on effectiveness CRD guidelines for those carrying out or commissioning reviews. CRD report no 4. York: NHS Centre for Reviews and Dissemination, University of York, 1996.
5   Chalmers I, Haynes RB. Reporting, updating, and correcting systematic reviews of the effects of health care. In: Chalmers I, Altman DG, eds. Systematic reviews. London: BMJ Publishing Group 1995: 86-95.

6   Bero L, Rennie D. The Cochrane Collaboration: preparing, maintaining, and disseminating systematic reviews of the effects of health care. *JAMA* 1995; 274: 1935-38.

7   Huston P. The Cochrane Collaboration helping unravel tangled web woven by international research. *Can Med Assoc J* 1996; 154: 1389-92.

8   Sacks HS, Berrier J, Reitman D, Ancona-Berk VA, Chalmers TC. Meta-analyses of randomized controlled trials. *N Engl J Med* 1987; 316: 450-55.

9   Sacks HS, Reitman D, Pagano D, Kupelnick B. Meta-analysis: an update. *Mt Sinai J Med* 1996; 63: 216-24.

10   Mulrow CD, Oxman AD, eds. Cochrane Collaboration Handbook. In: The Cochrane Library [database on disk and CDROM]. Oxford: Cochrane Collaboration. Update Software: 1994, issue 4.

11   Oxman AD, Cook DJ, Guyatt GH, and the Evidence-Based Medicine Working Group. Users' guides to the medical literature: VI, how to use an overview. *JAMA* 1994; 272: 1367-71.

12   Klassen TP, Jadad AR, Moher D. Guides for reading and interpreting systematic reviews: 1, getting started. *Arch Pediatr Adolesc Med* 1998; 152: 700-04.

13   L'Abbé KA, Detsky AS, O'Rourke K. Meta-analysis in clinical research. *Ann Intern Med* 1987; 107: 224-33.

14   Olkin I. A critical look at some popular meta-analytic methods. *Am J Epidemiol* 1984; 140: 287-88.

15   Olkin I. Statistical and theoretical considerations in meta-analysis. *J Clin Epidemiol* 1995; 48: 133-46.

16   Guyatt GH, Sackett DL, Sinclair J, Hayward R, Cook DJ, Cook RJ. Users' guides to the medical literature: IX, a method for grading health care recommendations. *JAMA* 1995; 274: 1800-04.

17   Jadad AR, Cook DJ, Browman G. A guide to interpreting discordant systematic reviews. *Can Med Assoc J* 1997; 156: 1411-16.

18   LeLorier J, Gregroire G, Benhaddad A, Lapierre J, Derderian F. Discrepancies between meta-analyses and subsequent large randomized, controlled trials. *N Engl J Med* 1997; 337: 536-42.

19   Shea B, Dubé C, Moher D. Assessing the quality of reports of meta-analyses: a systematic review of scales and checklists. In: Egger M, Davey Smith G, Altman DG, eds. Systematic reviews, 2nd edn. London: BMJ Publishing Group (in press).

20   The Standards of Reporting Trials Group. A proposal for structured reporting of randomized controlled trials. *JAMA* 1994; 272: 1926-31.

21   The Asilomar Working Group on Recommendations for Reporting of Clinical Trials in the Biomedical Literature. Checklist of information for inclusion in reports of clinical trials. *Ann Intern Med* 1996; 124: 741-43.

22   Begg C, Cho M, Eastwood S, et al. Improving the quality of reporting of randomized controlled trials: the CONSORT statement. *JAMA* 1996; 276: 637-39.

23   The Cochrane Library [database on disk and CDROM]. Oxford: Cochrane Collaboration. Update Software, 1996, issue 3.

24   Dickersin K, Scherer R, Lefebvre C. Identifying relevant studies for systematic reviews. *BMJ* 1994; 309: 1286-91.

25   Whitman N. The Delphi technique as an alternative for committee meetings. *J Nurs Educ* 1990; 29: 377-79.

26   Dickersin K, Higgins K, Meinert CL. Identification of meta-analyses: the need for standard terminology. *Control Clin Trials* 1990; 11: 52-66.

27   Taddio A, Pain T, Fassos FF, Boon H, Illersich AL, Einarson TR: Quality of nonstructured and structured abstracts of original research articles in the British Medical Journal, the Canadian Medical Association Journal and the Journal of the American Medical Association. *Can Med Assoc J* 1994; 150: 1611-15.

28   Tramér M, Reynolds DJM, Moore RA, McQuay HJ. Impact of covert duplicate publication on meta-analysis: a case study. *BMJ* 1997; 315: 635-40.

29   McAuley L, Moher D, Tugwell P. The influence of grey literature on meta-analysis. MSc Thesis: University of Ottawa, 1999.

30   Moher D, Pham B, Klassen TP, et al. Does the language of publication of reports of randomized trials influence the estimates of intervention effectiveness reported in meta-analyses? 6th Cochrane Colloquium; 1998.

31   Egger M, Zellweger-Zahner T, Schneider M, Junker C, Lengeler C, Antes G. Language bias in randomised controlled trials published in English and German. *Lancet* 1997; 350: 326-29.

32   Khan KS, Daya S, Collins JA, Walter S. Empirical evidence of bias in infertility research: overestimation of treatment effect in crossover trials using pregnancy as the outcome measure. *Fertil Steril* 1996; 65: 939-45.

33   Schulz KF, Chalmers I, Hayes RJ, Altman DG. Empirical evidence of bias: dimensions of methodological quality associated with estimates of treatment effects in controlled trials. *JAMA* 1995; 273: 408-12.

34   Moher D, Pham B, Jones A, et al. Does the quality of reports of randomised trials affect estimates of intervention efficacy reported in meta-analyses? *Lancet* 1998; 352: 609-13.

35   Jadad AR, Moore RA, Carroll D, et al. Assessing the quality of reports of randomized clinical trials: is blinding necessary? *Control Clin Trials* 1996; 17: 1-12.

36   Berlin JA on behalf of the University of Pennsylvania meta-analysis blinding study group. Does blinding of readers affect the results of meta-analyses? *Lancet* 1997; 350: 185-86.

37   Barnes DE, Bero LA. Why review articles on the health effects of passive smoking reach different conclusions. *JAMA* 1998; 279: 1566-70.

38   Thompson SG. Why sources of heterogeneity in meta-analysis should be investigated. *BMJ* 1994; 309: 1351-55.

39   Simes RJ. Publication bias: the case for an international registry of clinical trials. *J Clin Oncol* 1986; 4: 1529-41.

40   Sterling TD, Rosenbaum WL, Weinkam JJ. Publication decisions revisited: the effect of the outcome of statistical tests on the decision to publish and vice versa. *Am Statist* 1995; 49: 108-12.

41   Dickersin K, Min YI. NIH clinical trials and publication bias. *Online J Curr Clin Trials* 1993: April 28; doc no 50.

42   Easterbrook PJ, Berlin JA, Gopalan R, Matthews DR. Publication bias in clinical research. *Lancet* 1991; 337: 867-72.

43   Cook DJ, Guyatt GH, Ryan G, et al. Should unpublished data be included in meta-analyses? Current convictions and controversies. *JAMA* 1993; 269: 2749-53.

44   Smith ML. Publication bias and meta-analysis. *Eval Educ* 1980; 4: 22-24.

45   Moher D, Fortin P, Jadad AR, et al. Completeness of reporting of trials published in languages other than English: implications for conduct and reporting of systematic reviews. *Lancet* 1996; 347: 363-66.

46   Vickers A, Goyal N, Harland R, Rees R. Do certain countries produce only positive results? A systematic review of controlled trials. *Control Clin Trials* 1998; 19: 159-66.

47   Kennedy E, Song F, Hunter R, Clark A, Gilbody S. Risperidone versus typical antipsychotic medication for schizophrenia (Cochrane Review). In: Cochrane Library, issue 3. Oxford: Update Software, 1999.

48   Davies A, Adena MA, Keks NA, Catts SV, Lambert T, Schweitzer I. Risperidone versus haloperidol: I, meta-analysis of efficacy and safety. *Clin Ther* 1998; 20: 58-71.

49   Leucht S, Pitschel-Walz G, Abraham D, Kissling W. Efficacy and extrapyramidal side-effects of the new antipsychotics olanzapine, quetiapine, risperidone, and sertindole compared to conventional antipsychotics and placebo: a meta-analysis of randomized controlled trials. *Schizophrenia Res* 1999; 35: 51-68.

Appendix III

The CONSORT statement: revised recommendations for improving the quality of reports of parallel-group randomised trials

The CONSORT Group

David Moher, Kenneth F Schulz, Douglas G Altman,
for the CONSORT Group*
*Other members listed at end of paper

Reproduced with the kind permission
of The Lancet 2001; 357: 1191-94.

University of Ottawa, Thomas C Chalmers Centre for Systematic Reviews, Ottawa, Ontario, Canada (D Moher MSc); Family Health International and Department of Obstetrics and Gynecology, School of Medicine, University of North Carolina at Chapel Hill, NC, USA (K F Schulz PhD); and ICRF Medical Statistics Group and Centre for Statistics in Medicine, Institute of Health Sciences, Oxford, UK (D G Altman DSc)

Correspondence to: Dr Leah Lepage, Thomas C Chalmers Centre for Systematic Reviews, Children's Hospital of Eastern Ontario Research Institute, Room R235, 401 Smyth Road, Ottawa, Ontario K1H 8L1, Canada (e-mail:llepage@uottawa.ca)

To comprehend the results of a randomised controlled trial (RCT), readers must understand its design, conduct, analysis, and interpretation. That goal can be achieved only through total transparency from authors. Despite several decades of educational efforts, the reporting of RCTs needs improvement. Investigators and editors developed the original CONSORT (Consolidated Standards of Reporting Trials) statement to help authors improve reporting by use of a checklist and flow diagram. The revised CONSORT statement presented here incorporates new evidence and addresses some criticisms of the original statement. The checklist items pertain to the content of the Title, Abstract, Introduction, Methods, Results, and Discussion. The revised checklist includes 22 items selected because empirical evidence indicates that not reporting this information is associated with biased estimates of treatment effect, or because the information is essential to judge the reliability or relevance of the findings. We intended the flow diagram to depict the passage of participants through an RCT. The revised flow diagram depicts information from four stages of a trial (enrolment, intervention allocation, follow-up, and analysis). The diagram explicitly shows the number of participants, for each intervention group, included in the primary data analysis. Inclusion of these numbers allows the reader to judge whether the authors have done an intention-to-treat analysis. In sum, the CONSORT statement is intended to improve the reporting of an RCT, enabling readers to understand a trial's conduct and to assess the validity of its results.

A report of a randomised controlled trial (RCT) should convey to the reader, in a transparent manner, why the study was undertaken, and how it was conducted and analysed. Inadequately reported randomisation, for example, has been associated with bias in estimating the effectiveness of interventions.[1,2] To assess the strengths and limitations of an RCT, readers need and deserve to know the quality of its methods.

Despite several decades of educational efforts, RCTs are still not being reported adequately.[3-6] For example, a review[5] of 122 recently published RCTs that assessed the effectiveness of selective serotonin reuptake inhibitors as a first-line management strategy for depression found that only one paper described randomisation adequately. Inadequate reporting makes the interpretation of RCTs difficult, if not impossible. Moreover, inadequate reporting borders on unethical practice when biased results receive false credibility.

History of CONSORT

In the mid-1990s, two independent initiatives to improve the quality of reports of RCTs led to the publication of the CONSORT statement,[7] which was developed by an international group of clinical trialists, statisticians, epidemiologists, and biomedical editors. CONSORT has been supported by a growing number of medical and health-care journals[8-11] and editorial groups, including the International Committee of Medical Journal Editors (ICMJE, The Vancouver Group),[12] the Council of Science Editors (CSE), and the World Association of Medical Editors (WAME). CONSORT is published in Dutch, English, French, German, Japanese, and Spanish. It can be accessed together with other information about the CONSORT group on the internet.[13]

The CONSORT statement consists of a checklist and flow diagram for reporting an RCT. For convenience, the checklist and diagram together are called simply CONSORT. They are primarily intended for use in writing, reviewing, or assessing reports of simple two-group parallel RCTs.

Preliminary data indicate that the use of CONSORT does indeed help to improve the quality of reports of RCTs.[14,15] In an assessment[14] of 71 RCTs, published in three journals in 1994, allocation concealment was not clearly reported in 43 (61%) of the trials. 4 years later, after these three journals required that authors reporting an RCT use CONSORT, the proportion of papers in which allocation concealment was not clearly reported had dropped to 30 of 77 (39%, mean difference -22% [95% CI -38 to -6]).

The usefulness of CONSORT is increased by continuous monitoring of biomedical publications, which allows it to be modified dependent on the merits of maintaining or dropping current items, and including new items. For example, when Meinert[16] observed that the flow diagram did not provide important information about the number of participants who entered each phase of an RCT (i.e. enrolment, treatment allocation, follow-up, and data analysis), the diagram could be modified to accommodate the information. The checklist is similarly flexible.

This iterative process makes the CONSORT statement a continually evolving instrument. Although participants in the CONSORT group and their degree of involvement vary over time, members meet regularly to review the need to refine CONSORT. At the 1999 meeting, the participants decided to revise the original statement. This report reflects changes determined by consensus of the CONSORT group, partly in response to emerging evidence on the importance of various elements of RCTs.

Revision of the CONSORT statement

13 members of the CONSORT group met in May, 1999, with the main objective of revising the original CONSORT checklist and flow diagram, as needed. The group discussed the merits of including each item in the light of current evidence. As in developing the original CONSORT statement, our intention was to keep only those items

deemed fundamental to reporting standards for an RCT. Some items not regarded as essential could well be highly desirable and should still be included in an RCT report even though they are not included in CONSORT. Such items include approval of an institutional ethics review board, sources of funding for the trial, and a trial registry number - e.g. the International Standard Randomized Controlled Trial Number (ISRCTN) used to register the RCT at its inception.[17]

Shortly after the meeting, a revised version of the checklist was circulated to the group for additional comments and feedback. Revisions to the flow diagram were similarly made. All these changes were discussed when CONSORT participants met in May, 2000, and the revised statement was finalised shortly afterwards.

The revised CONSORT statement includes a 22-item checklist (table) and a flow diagram (figure). Its main aim is to help authors improve the quality of reports of simple two-group parallel RCTs. However, the basic philosophy underlying the development of the statement can be applied to any design. In this respect, additional statements for other designs will be forthcoming from the group. CONSORT can also be used by peer reviewers and editors to identify reports with inadequate description of trials and those with potentially biased results.[1,2]

During the 1999 meeting, the group also discussed the benefits of developing an explanatory document to improve the use and dissemination of CONSORT. The document is patterned on reporting of statistical aspects of clinical research,[18] and was developed to help facilitate the recommendations of the ICMJE's Uniform Requirements for Manuscripts Submitted to Biomedical Journals. Three members of the CONSORT group, with assistance from members on some checklist items, drafted an explanation and elaboration document. That document[19] was circulated to the group for additions and revisions and was last revised after review at the latest CONSORT group meeting.

Checklist of items to include when reporting a randomised trial

	Item number	Descriptor	Reported on page number
Title and abstract	1	How participants were allocated to interventions (e.g. 'random allocation', 'randomised', or 'randomly assigned').	
Introduction			
Background	2	Scientified background and explanation of rationale.	
Methods			
Participants	3	Eligibility criteria for participants and the settings and locations where the data were collected.	
Interventions	4	Precise details of the interventions intended for each group and how and when they were actually administered.	
Objectives	5	Specific objectives and hypotheses.	
Outcomes	6	Clearly defined primary and secondary outcome measures and, when applicable, any methods used to enhance the quality of measurements (e.g. multiple observations, training of assessors, &c).	
Sample size	7	How sample size was determined and, when applicable, explanation of any interim analyses and stopping rules.	
Randomisation			
Sequence generation	8	Method used to generate the random allocation sequence, including details of any restriction (e.g. blocking, stratification).	
Allocation concealment	9	Method used to implement the random allocation sequence (e.g. numbered containers or central telephone), clarifying whether the sequence was concealed until interventions were assigned.	
Implementation	10	Who generated the allocation sequence, who enrolled participants, and who assigned participants to their groups.	
Blinding (masking)	11	Whether or not participants, those administering the interventions, and those assessing the outcomes were aware of group assignment. If not, how the success of masking was assessed.	
Statistical methods	12	Statistical methods used to compare groups for primary outcome(s); methods for additional analyses, such as subgroup analyses and adjusted analyses.	

	Item number	Descriptor	Reported on page number
Results			
Participant flow	13	Flow of participants through each stage (a diagram is strongly recommended). Specifically, for each group, report the numbers of participants randomly assigned, receiving intended treatment, completing the study protocol, and analysed for the primary outcome. Describe protocol deviations from study as planned, together with reasons.	
Recruitment	14	Dates defining the periods of recruitment and follow-up.	
Baseline data	15	Baseline demographic and clinical characteristics of each group.	
Numbers analysed	16	Number of participants (denominator) in each group included in each analysis and whether the analysis was by 'intention to treat'. State the results in absolute numbers when feasible (e.g. 10/20, not 50%).	
Outcomes and estimation	17	For each primary and secondary outcome, a summary of results for each group, and the estimated effect size and its precision (e.g. 95% CI).	
Ancillary analyses	18	Address multiplicity by reporting any other analyses performed, including subgroup analyses and adjusted analyses, indicating those prespecified and those exploratory.	
Adverse events	19	All important adverse events or side-effects in each intervention group.	
Discussion			
Interpretation	20	Interpretation of the results, taking into account study hypotheses, sources of potential bias or imprecision and the dangers associated with multiplicity of analyses and outcomes.	
Generalisability	21	Generalisability (external validity) of the trial findings.	
Overall evidence	22	General interpretation of the results in the context of current evidence.	

Flow diagram of the progress through the phases of a randomised trial

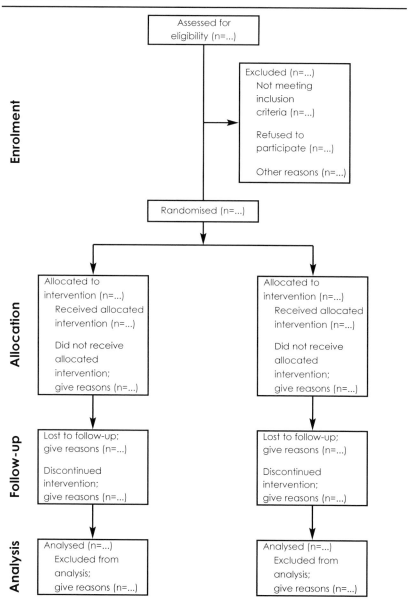

Changes to CONSORT

(1) In the revised checklist, a new column for 'Paper section and topic' integrates information from the 'Subheading' column that was contained in the original statement.

(2) The 'Was it reported?' column has been integrated into a 'reported on page number' column, as requested by some journals.

(3) Each item of the checklist is now numbered and the syntax and order have been revised to improve the flow of information.

(4) 'Title' and 'Abstract' are now combined in the first item.

(5) Although the content of the revised checklist is similar to the original, some items that were previously combined are now separate. For example, previously authors were asked to describe 'primary and secondary outcome(s) measure(s) and the minimum important difference(s), and indicate how the target sample size was projected'. In the new version, issues pertaining to outcomes (item 6) and sample size (item 7) are separate, enabling authors to be more explicit about each. Moreover, some items request additional information. For example, for outcomes, authors are asked to report any methods used to improve the quality of measurements, such as multiple observations.

(6) The item asking for the unit of randomisation (e.g. cluster) has been dropped because specific checklists have been developed for reporting cluster RCTs[20] and other design types[13] since publication of the original checklist.

(7) Whenever possible, new evidence is incorporated into the revised checklist. For example, authors are asked to be explicit about whether the analysis reported is by intention to treat (item 16). This request is based partly on the observations[21] that authors do not adequately describe and apply intention-to-treat analysis, and that reports not

providing this information are less likely to provide other relevant information such as losses to follow-up.[22]

(8) The revised flow diagram depicts information from four stages of a trial (enrolment, intervention allocation, follow-up, and analysis). The revised diagram explicitly shows the number of participants, for each intervention group, included in the primary data analysis. Inclusion of these numbers lets the reader know whether the authors have done an intention-to-treat analysis.[21-23] Because some of the information might not always be known, and to accommodate other information, the structure of the flow diagram might need to be modified for a particular trial. Inclusion of the participant flow diagram in the report is strongly recommended but might be unnecessary for simple trials such as those without any participant withdrawals or dropouts.

Discussion

Specifically developed to guide authors about how to improve the quality of reporting of simple two-group parallel RCTs, CONSORT encourages transparency with reporting of the methods and results so that reports of RCTs can be interpreted readily and accurately. However, CONSORT does not address other facets of reporting that also require attention, such as scientific content and readability of RCT reports. Some authors in their enthusiasm to use CONSORT have modified the checklist.[24] We recommend against such modifications because they could be based on a different process from the one used by the CONSORT group.

The use of CONSORT seems to reduce, if not eliminate, inadequate reporting of RCTs.[14,15] Potentially, the use of CONSORT should positively influence the manner in which RCTs are conducted. Granting agencies have noted this potential relation, and in at least one case[25] have encouraged researchers to consider in their application how they have dealt with the CONSORT items.

The evidence-based approach used to develop CONSORT has also been used to develop standards for reporting meta-analyses of randomised trials,[26] meta-analyses of observational studies,[27] and diagnostic studies (Jeroen Lijmer, personal communication). Health economists have also started to develop reporting standards[28] to help to improve the quality of their reports.[29] The intent of all these initiatives is to improve the quality of reporting of biomedical research,[30] and by doing so, to bring about more effective health care.

The revised CONSORT statement will replace the original one in the journals and groups that already support it. Journals that do not yet support CONSORT may do so by registering on the CONSORT website.[13] To convey to authors the importance of improved quality in the reporting of RCTs, we encourage supporting journals to reference the revised CONSORT statement and the CONSORT internet address in their Instructions to Contributors. Since the journals publishing the revised CONSORT statement have waived copyright protection, CONSORT is now widely accessible to the biomedical community. The CONSORT checklist and flow diagram can also be accessed at the CONSORT website.

A lack of clarification of the meaning and rationale for each checklist item in the original CONSORT statement has been remedied with the development of the CONSORT explanation and elaboration document,[19] which can also be found on the CONSORT website. This document reports the evidence on which the checklist items are based, including the references, which had annotated the checklist items in the previous version. We also encourage journals to include reference to this document in their Instructions to Contributors.

Emphasising the evolving nature of CONSORT, the CONSORT group invites readers to comment on the updated checklist and flow diagram through the CONSORT website.[13] Comments and suggestions will be collated and considered at the next meeting of the group in 2001.

279

Contributors

David Moher, Ken Schulz, and Doug Altman participated in regular conference calls, identified participants, participated in the CONSORT meetings, and drafted the paper. David Moher and Leah Lepage planned the CONSORT meetings, identified and secured funding, invited the participants, and planned the meeting agenda. The members of the CONSORT group listed below attended the CONSORT meetings and provided input towards the revised checklist, flow diagram, and text.

The CONSORT group

Frank Davidoff (*Annals of Internal Medicine*, Philadelphia, PA, USA); Susan Eastwood (University of California at San Francisco, CA, USA); Matthias Egger (Department of Social Medicine, University of Bristol, UK); Diana Elbourne (London School of Hygiene and Tropical Medicine, London, UK); Peter Gøtzsche (Nordic Cochrane Centre, Copenhagen, Denmark); Sylvan B Green (School of Medicine, Case Western Reserve University, Cleveland, OH, USA); Leni Grossman (Merck & Co, Whitehouse Station, NJ, USA); Barbara S Hawkins (Wilmer Ophthal-mological Institute, Johns Hopkins University, (Baltimore, MD, USA); Richard Horton (*The Lancet*, London, UK); Wayne B Jonas (Uniformed Services University of the Health Sciences, Bethesda, MD); Terry Klassen (Department of Pediatrics, University of Alberta, Edmonton, Alberta, Canada); Leah Lepage (Thomas C Chalmers Centre for Systematic Reviews, Ottawa, Ontario, Canada); Thomas Lang (Tom Lang Communications, Lakewood, OH, USA); Jeroen Lijmer (Department of Clinical Epidemiology, University of Amsterdam, Netherlands); Rick Malone (TAP Pharmaceuticals, Lake Forest, IL, USA); Curtis L Meinert (Johns Hopkins University, Baltimore, MD); Mary Mosley (Life Science Publishing, Tokyo, Japan); Stuart Pocock (London School of Hygiene and Tropical Medicine, London); Drummond Rennie (*Journal of the American Medical Association*, Chicago, IL); David S Riley

(University of New Mexico Medical School, Santa Fe, NM, USA); Roberta W Scherer (Epidemiology & Preventive Medicine, University of Maryland School of Medicine, Baltimore, MD); Ida Sim (University of California at San Francisco, CA); Donna Stroup (Epidemiology Program Office, Centers for Disease Control and Prevention, Atlanta, GA, USA).

Acknowledgments

The effort to improve the reporting of randomised trials, from its beginnings with the Standards of Reporting Trials (SORT) group to the current activities of the Consolidated Standards of Reporting Trials (CONSORT) group, has involved many people around the globe. We thank Leah Lepage for keeping everybody all lined up and moving in the same direction. Financial support to convene meetings of the CONSORT group was provided in part by Abbott Laboratories, American College of Physicians, GlaxoWellcome, *The Lancet*, Merck, the Canadian Institutes for Health Research, National Library of Medicine, and TAP Pharmaceuticals.

References

1   Schulz KF, Chalmers I, Hayes RJ, Altman DG. Empirical evidence of bias: dimensions of methodological quality associated with estimates of treatment effects in controlled trials. *JAMA* 1995; 273: 408-12.

2   Moher D, Pham B, Jones A, et al. Does the quality of reports of randomised trials affect estimates of intervention efficacy reported in meta-analyses? *Lancet* 1998; 352: 609-13.

3   Jadad AR, Boyle M, Cunningham C, Kim M, Schachar R. Treatment of attention deficit/hyperactivity disorder: evidence report/technology assessment no 11. Hamilton: McMaster University, 2000.

4   Thornley B, Adams CE. Content and quality of 2000 controlled trials in schizophrenia over 50 years. *BMJ* 1998; 317: 1181-84.

5   Hotopf M, Lewis G, Normand C. Putting trials on trial - the costs and consequences of small trials in depression: a systematic review of methodology. *J Epidemiol Community Health* 1997; 51: 354-58.

6   Dickinson K, Bunn F, Wentz R, Edwards P, Roberts I. Size and quality of randomised controlled trials in head injury: review of published studies. *BMJ* 2000; 320: 1308-11.

7   Begg CB, Cho MK, Eastwood S, et al. Improving the quality of reporting of randomized controlled trials: the CONSORT statement. *JAMA* 1996; 276: 637-39.

8   Freemantle N, Mason JM, Haines A, Eccles MP. CONSORT: an important step toward evidence-based health care. *Ann Intern Med* 1997; 126: 81-83.

9   Altman DG. Better reporting of randomized controlled trials: the CONSORT statement. *BMJ* 1996; 313: 570-71.

10 Schulz KF. The quest for unbiased research: randomized clinical trials and the CONSORT reporting guidelines. *Ann Neurol* 1997; 41: 569-73.

11 Huston P. Hoey J. CMAJ endorses the CONSORT statement. *Can Med Assoc J* 1996; 155: 1277-79.

12 Davidoff F. News from the International Committee of Medical Journal Editors. *Ann Intern Med* 2000; 133: 229-31.

13 www.consort-statement.org (accessed Feb 15, 2001).

14 Moher D, Jones A, Lepage L, for the CONSORT Group. Use of CONSORT statement and quality of reports of randomized trials: a comparative before and after evaluation? *JAMA* (in press).

15 Egger M, Juni P, Bartiett C, for the CONSORT Group. The value of patient flow charts in reports of randomized controlled trials: bibliographic study. *JAMA* (in press).

16 Meinert CL. Beyond CONSORT: need for improved reporting standards for clinical trials. *JAMA* 1998; 279: 1487-89.

17 Chalmers I. Current Controlled Trials: an opportunity to help improve the quality of clinical research. *Curr Control Trials Cardiovasc Med* 2000; 1: 3-8.

18 Bailer JC III, Mosteller F. Guidelines for statistical reporting in articles for medical journals: amplifications and explanations. *Ann Intern Med* 1988; 108: 266-73.

19 Altman DG, Schulz KF, Moher D, et al, for the CONSORT group. The revised CONSORT statement for reporting randomized trials: explanation and elaboration. *Ann Intern Med* 2001; 134: 663-94.

20 Elbourne DR, Campbell MK. Extending the CONSORT statement to cluster randomised trials: for discussion. *Stat Med* (in press).

21 Hollis S, Campbell F. What is meant by intention-to-treat analysis? Survey of published randomized controlled trials. *BMJ* 1999; 319: 670-74.

22 Ruiz-Canela M. Martinez-Gonzalez MA, de Irala-Estevez J. Intention-to-treat analysis is related to methodological quality. *BMJ* 2000; 320: 1007.

23 Lee YJ, Ellenberg JH, Hirtz DG, Nelson KB. Analysis of clinical trials by treatment actually received: is it really an option? *Stat Med* 1991; 10: 1595-605.

24 Bentzen SM. Towards evidence based radiation oncology: improving the design, analysis, and reporting of clinical outcome studies in radiotherapy. *Radiother Oncol* 1998; 46: 5-18.

25 O'Toole LB. MRC uses checklist similar to CONSORT's. *BMJ* 1997; 314: 1127.

26 Moher D, Cook DJ, Eastwood S, Olkin I, Rennie D, Stroup DF, for the QUOROM group. Improving the quality of reports of meta-analyses of randomised controlled trials: the QUOROM statement. *Lancet* 1999; 354: 1896-900.

27 Stroup DF, Berlin IA, Morton SC, et al. Meta-analysis of observational studies in epidemiology: a proposal for reporting. *JAMA* 2000; 283: 2008-12.

28 Siegel IE, Weinstein MC, Russell LB, Gold MR. Recommendations for reporting cost-effectiveness analysis. *JAMA* 1996; 276: 1339-41.

29 Neumann PJ, Stone PW, Chapman RH, Sandberg EA, Bell CM. The quality of reporting in published cost-utility analyses, 1976-1997. *Ann Intern Med* 2000; 132: 964-72.

30 Altman DG. The scandal of poor medical research. *BMJ* 1994; 308: 283-84.

Appendix
III

Appendix IV

Consensus statement on submission and publication of manuscripts

Surgery 2001; 129 (6): 662-3

Increasing problems of duplicate and fraudulent submissions and publications have prompted the undersigned editors of surgical journals to support these overall principles of publication.

Duplicate submission and publication

In general, if a manuscript has been peer-reviewed and published, any subsequent publication is duplication. Exceptions to this general rule may be:

a) Prior publication in meeting program abstract booklets or expanded abstracts such as those published by the *Surgical Forum* of the American College of Surgeons or *Transplantation Proceedings*. However, these must be referenced in the final manuscript.

b) A manuscript that extends an original database (a good rule might be expansion by 50% or more) or that analyzes the original database in a different way in order to prove or disprove a different hypothesis. Previous manuscripts reporting the original database must, however, be referenced.

c) Manuscripts that have been published originally in non-English language journals, provided that the prior publication is clearly indicated on the English language submission and referenced in the manuscript. In some circumstances, permission to publish may need to be obtained from the non-English language journal.

For example, any submission duplicating material previously published in full in 'Proceedings' or book chapters is considered duplicate unless the exceptions in a) above apply. Similarly, manuscripts dealing with subgroups of data (i.e. patients) that have previously been analyzed, discussed, and published as a larger group are considered duplicate unless b) above applies.

The Internet raises special concerns. If data has previously appeared on the Internet, submission of that data for publication is considered duplication. If Internet publication follows journal publication, the journal publication should be clearly referenced. Some journals may provide early Internet publication of accepted peer-reviewed papers that are subsequently published in that journal. This does not constitute duplication if both manuscripts are identical and covered by the same single copyright.

Fraudulent publication

The following activities are examples of fraudulent publication practices:

a) Wilful and knowing submissions of false data for publication.

b) Submission of data from sources not the author's (or authors') own.

c) Falsely certifying that the submitted work is original and has not been submitted to, or accepted by, another journal.

d) Sponsoring or vouching for a manuscript containing data over which the sponsor has no control or knowledge.

e) Allowing one's name to appear as an author without having contributed significantly to the study.

f) Adding an author's name to a manuscript to which he/she has not contributed or reviewed or agreed to in its current form.

g) Flagrant omission of reference to work of other investigators, which established their priority.

h) Falsification of any item on the copyright form.

i) Failure to disclose potential conflict of interest with a sponsoring agency.

While not intended as an all-inclusive document, these examples and guidelines should alert authors to potential problems that should be avoided when they are considering submission of a manuscript to a peer-reviewed journal.

American Journal of Surgery	Hiram C. Polk, Jr, MD
American Surgeon	Talmadge A. Bowden, Jr, MD
Annals of Surgery	Layton F. Rikkers, MD
Annals of Surgical Oncology	Charles M. Balch, MD
Current Surgery	Walter J. Pories, MD
Digestive Surgery	Eduard H. Farthmann, MD
	Markus W. Büchler, MD
Diseases of the Colon and Rectum	Victor Fazio, MD
Journal of the American College of Surgeons	Seymour Schwartz, MD
Journal of Gastrointestinal Surgery	John L. Cameron, MD
	Keith A. Kelly, MD
Journal of Japan Medical Association	Yasuo Idezuki, MD
Journal of Japan Society for Endoscopic Surgery	Yasuo Idezuki, MD
Journal of Japan Surgical Association	Yasuo Idezuki, MD
Journal of Pediatric Surgery	Jay Grosfeld, MD
Journal of Surgical Research	Wiley W. Souba, MD
	David W. McFadden, MD
Journal of Thoracic and Cardiovascular Surgery	Andrew S. Wechsler, MD
Journal of Vascular Surgery	Robert B. Rutherford, MD
	K. Wayne Johnston, MD
Journal of Parenteral and Enteral Nutrition	Danny O. Jacobs, MD
Journal of Trauma	Basil A. Pruitt, Jr, MD
Surgery	Andrew L. Warshaw, MD
	Michael Sarr, MD
Surgical Endoscopy	Bruce V. MacFadyen, Jr, MD
	Sir Alfred Cuschieri, MD
Surgical Laparoscopy, Endoscopy and	
Percutaneous Techniques	Carol E. H. Scott-Conner, MD, PhD
	Maurice Arregui, MD
World Journal of Surgery	Ronald K. Tompkins, MD
Zentralblatt für Chirurgie	Albrecht Encke, MD